The AMDP-System in Pharmacopsychiatry

Modern Problems of Pharmacopsychiatry

Vol. 20

Series Editors
T.A. Ban, Nashville, Tenn.; *F.A. Freyhan*†, Washington, D.C.;
P. Pichot, Paris, and *W. Pöldinger,* Wil/St. Gallen

KARGER

S. Karger · Basel · München · Paris · London · New York · Tokyo · Sydney

The AMDP-System in Pharmacopsychiatry

Volume Editors
D. Bobon, Liège; *U. Baumann,* Salzburg; *J. Angst,* Zürich;
H. Helmchen, Berlin; *H. Hippius,* Munich

27 figures and 84 tables, 1983

KARGER

S. Karger · Basel · München · Paris · London · New York · Tokyo · Sydney

Modern Problems of Pharmacopsychiatry

National Library of Medicine, Cataloging in Publication
The AMDP-system in pharmacopsychiatry
Volume editors, D. Bobon ... [et al.]. – Basel, New York, Karger, 1983.
(Modern problems of pharmacopsychiatry, v. 20)
1. Mental Disorders – diagnosis 2. Psychiatric Status Rating Scales 3. Psychotropic Drugs I. Bobon, D. II. Series
W1 MO168P v. 20 [WM 141 A4965]
ISBN 3-8055-3637-2

Drug Dosage

The authors and the publisher have exerted every effort to ensure that drug selection and dosage set forth in this text are in accord with current recommendations and practice at the time of publication. However, in view of ongoing research, changes in government regulations, and the constant flow of information relating to drug therapy and drug reactions, the reader is urged to check the package insert for each drug for any change in indications and dosage and for added warnings and precautions. This is particularly important when the recommended agent is a new and/or infrequently employed drug.

Printed in Switzerland by Meier+Cie AG Schaffhausen
ISBN 3-8055-3637-2

Contents

Validity and Sensitivity in Drug Trials

Appendix I

Appendix II

History and Description

Mod. Probl. Pharmacopsychiat., vol. 20, pp. 1–9 (Karger, Basel 1983)

The History of the AMDP-System

E. Fähndrich[a], *H. Helmchen*[a], *H. Hippius*[b],

[a]Department of Psychiatry, Free University of Berlin, Berlin, FRG;
[b]Department of Psychiatry, University, of Munich, Munich, FRG

The mode of action of neuroleptic therapy was discovered in France in 1952 with Chlorpromazine, which was then introduced into clinical psychiatry. Already within a few years neuroleptics had earned themselves a firm foothold in the whole world in psychiatric *therapy*. Furthermore, the discovery of the antipsychotic efficacy of Chlorpromazine became the starting point of modern psychopharmacology as a *science*. With the cooperation of various other disciplines of medical basic research (e.g. biochemistry, experimental neurophysiology, etiology, etc.) psychopharmacology has become as *neuropsychopharmacology* one of the most active areas of pharmacological *basic research*. Above all, clinical-psychiatric research has been given especially important impulses as far as the therapeutic application of psychotropic drugs is concerned.

Clinical pharmacology developed particularly fruitfully in psychiatry. A retrospect over the years since 1952 shows that with the development of practical pharmacopsychiatry a basis has been created for a modern psychiatric *therapy research*.

In German-speaking areas the Association for Methodology and Documentation in Psychiatry (AMP) system (the new abbreviation of which since 1978/79 is AMDP-System) has played an important part in the development of psychiatric research. In all clinics scientifically studying the therapeutic effects of Chlorpromazine since 1952, it was very soon necessary that such studies should be carried out using definite methods. On the one hand, this was based on the necessity to be able to compare the findings of one clinic with those of other clinics. On the other hand, shortly after the introduction of Chlorpromazine an ever-increasing number of potentially effective psychotropic drugs was developed, which of course needed to be compared with the older and already proven drugs. Also by this time the scientists from the different clinics were interested in performing therapy studies with the new psychotropic drugs with the participation of several clinics. It became obvious that these three intentions could only be fulfilled with the necessary reliability when definite and trustworthy methods were applied, which could be used by different investigators.

At the end of the 1950s five psychiatric university clinics in the FRG got together in a study group to work out such clinically applicable methods *(Bente,* Erlangen; *Heinrich,* Mainz; *Helmchen, Hippius,* Berlin; *Engelmeier,* Münster; *Schmitt,* Homburg/Saar). The aim of this collaboration was to set out a joint investigation procedure for these five clinics, which would be performed before, during and after treatment. At the beginning of this collaboration all five clinics were able to refer to their many years of practical experience with their own means of investigation – as for example, the reference to the 'Erlanger Pioneer Scale' developed by *Bente* for the Erlangen clinic. Having set up a combined investigation and documentation instrument for all participants, a few joint studies or 'multicenter trials' were carried out to test the practicability of this procedure and to characterize the mode of effect of various new psychotropic drugs. The resulting methodical knowledge obtained from these studies was first summarized by *Bente* et al. [1961].

In Switzerland there was a similar development. However, it was remarkable that unlike in Germany, all psychiatric university clinics participated right from the start and without exception (*Angst,* Zürich; *Cornu,* Bern; *Dick,* Geneva; *Heimann,* Lausanne; *Pöldinger,* Basel). The first results of this Swiss collaboration were published by *Angst* et al. [1964].

As far as application was concerned, the procedures of the Swiss and German clinics were very similar to each other. Unlike the very intense attempts of the English-speaking psychiatry at this period to develop so-called 'psychiatric rating scales' to comprehend and record either specific psychopathological syndromes (e.g. depression, anxiety), or an extensive psychopathological finding (e.g. In-Patient Multidimensional Psychiatric Scale, IMPS; Brief Psychiatric Rating Scale, BPRS), the aim of the German as well as the Swiss group was to comprehend and record an entire psychiatric finding with the inclusion of demographic and anamnestic data at the start of the investigation. Thus, it was clear that the Swiss and German groups would decide upon a further collaboration. This followed soon after in 1965 and occurred moreover with the participation of an Austrian university clinic (*Berner,* Vienna). Since an important aim of the collaboration lay in the comprehension and description of the *course of the illness,* especially under *treatment with psychotropic drugs,* scientists from the Swiss pharmaceutical industry (*Schmidlin and Weis,* Ciba-Geigy, Basel), who had already previously participated in the work of the Swiss clinics in the field of method development, joined the German-Swiss group.

From 1965 onwards the German-Swiss group, which had been formed in this way, called itself the *Arbeitsgemeinschaft für Methodik und Dokumentation in der Psychiatrie* – originally abbreviated as AMP (translated: Association for Methodology and Documentation in Psychiatry). Although the original abbreviation given to the association does not mention the concept 'documentation', this was unintentional. Even at the beginning, the importance of this methodical step of 'documentation' for the development of psychiatric research should be emphasized.

Since 1965 it has been the main endeavor of the AMP to identify psychiatrically relevant data, to record them and thus to make them available for statistical processing. In this way such changes in symptoms over a period of time, i.e. in their course and usually as a consequence of therapeutic measures, should be mathematically exhibited. In order that the system was a success, the first step, namely an accurate collection of data and its documentation, was of an utmost importance. The development of the documentation system was time-consuming; 2 years after the foundation of the association, the common system was made public [*Angst* et al., 1967]; it was then named AMP [*Angst* et al., 1969]. The first edition of the Manual appeared six years after the German-Swiss merging [*Scharfetter,* 1971].

Originally, the AMP documentation system consisted of four opscan sheets, which could be converted into punch cards by optical readers. The AMP-System was different from other psychiatric documentation systems, in that not only were psychiatrically relevant symptoms and side-effects of psychotropic drugs recorded but also biographical data and incidents immediately prior to the disease were noted. For example, the documentation of the history (AMP sheet 1) contained details of the patient's family (e.g. number of brothers and sisters, position of the patient in the line of brothers and sisters, details of patient's own children, etc.). Besides this, details on the ability of verbal expression, career training as well as the career position at the time of admission and details about the patient's attitude towards his career were recorded.

The disease anamnesis (AMP sheet 2) covered the psychiatric features in the biological family of the patient, disorders in his familial situation during childhood (e.g. divorce of the parents, possible stays at foster home, etc.) and trends in his psychosocial development (e.g. tendencies towards degeneration, drug abuse, criminality or possible suicide attempts). Any psychic disorders which had occurred earlier were documented as well as any previous incidents which, in the opinion of the doctor, were connected with the present illness. Furthermore, past treatments with psychotropic drugs or electroshock therapy and its efficacy as well as diagnosis according to the International Classification of Diseases (ICD) were recorded. The core of the AMP-System lay in the sheet 'psychopathological symptoms' (previously sheet 3, now 4) and 'somatic signs' (previously sheet 4, now 5).

The symptoms contained in the characteristic catalogue were derived from the classic descriptive psychopathology and were therefore – at least in the German-speaking psychiatry – not controversial and of general use. In a 'test of the objectivity', which took place in the so-called 'Homburg experiment' [*Pöldinger,* 1969] before the publication of the sheets, the representatives of all eleven participating clinics attempted a first interrater reliability test. This experiment's task was to put to test the scientific content of the clinical language used. It became vital to define the various stages of importance in deciding on the existence or non-existence of a particular trait. One of the main results of this 'Homburg experiment' proved that to test concordance, the definite stages are of great importance in leading to the individual assertions [*Pöldinger,* 1969]. The logic model of this stage of decision is shown in figure 1. Apart from this, the Homburg symposium illustrated the necessity to produce a manual for the operation of the system and for the definition of the items. This manual appeared 2 years later [*Scharfetter,* 1971].

One of the difficulties in developing the AMP-System lay in defining the formal precision of the documentation system. Above all, it was the group's opinion that they had developed an instrument which possessed an apparent reliability similar to a psychological test procedure. *Heimann* et al. [1976] wrote in this context: 'Our group has seen the problem firstly in analogy to experimental psychology, as that of the reliabilty of examining instruments and correspondingly has undertaken investigations towards solving this problem. Not until we started elaborating logically and with regard to the contents of the achieved results did we realize that we were not dealing with a test procedure with a given reliability,

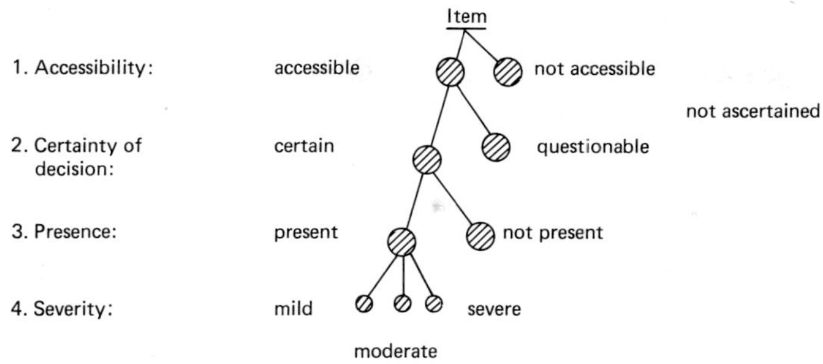

Fig. 1. Decision tree.

but with a clinical documentation procedure, whose objectivity can be arbitrarily perfected by a systematical and controlled training. Once achieved, synchronization coefficients do not prove the instrument as such, but prove the research group working with the documentation system, whose mutuality in the observation language is identified by these coefficients.'

This means that each group working with the AMP-System must state its own interrater reliability. A satisfactory result can only be achieved by constant, communal training, which as a rule is nowadays made with the aid of video films and subsequent discussion of the individual items [*Busch* et al., 1975; *von Cranach and Strauss,* 1977].

A first interrater reliability trial was carried out at the Berlin University Clinic by *Gebhardt and Helmchen* [1973]. Here it was possible to show that this reliability does not depend on the general clinical-psychiatric experience of the various investigators, but is clearly dependent on the confidence of the latter in practical use of the AMP-System.

Thus, in 1974 in Berlin at the First AMP Symposium the influence of the training on the interrater reliability was examined [*Busch* et al., 1975]. For this experiment 21 psychiatrists from 10 different clinics in Austria, Switzerland, Belgium and Germany were shown video films of psychiatric exploration (the length of the individual films was on average 30 minutes). After projection of the first video film each participant had to record his observations on the AMP sheet 'psychopathological symptoms'. The video film was *not* discussed afterwards. For the following 6 films each participant once again had to submit his finding to the AMP sheet without discussing his opinions with the other investigators.

Following this individual and independent documentation, each of the films was discussed item by item by all participants and this discussion was continued until all participants were in agreement with each others' findings.

At the end of the seminar, which lasted one and a half days, the first video film was shown again and recorded again with the AMP sheet 'psychopathological symptoms'. Then the results of both ratings were compared. The comparison of the documentation of findings from this video film shown both at the beginning and end of the training seminar was made in order to test whether combined training leads to a better unity between psychiatrists with completely different psychiatric experience and from differing schools of thought as far as the AMP items are concerned. In order to unify the judgement, it was intended to decrease the deviation of the individual symptoms and to increase the similarity of the profile. In the formation of extreme groups 11 items in the first rating could be distinguished by a non-coincidentally large deviation; however, in the control rating this was then only 6. The number of items, which showed a slight or no deviation at all, i.e. where there was a large agreement, rose from 65 to 76. Thus, in the course of the training the items over which one was in agreement increased, whilst those over which one was not in agreement decreased.

In the first years the AMP-System was predominantly used in the scientific study of the effect of psychotropic drugs [*Angst and Woggon,* this volume]. This required a corresponding organization of data and the development of differential evaluation programs [*Stassen* et al., this volume].

The work with the AMP-System soon meant that this comprehensive documentation system was not only used to test the efficacy of drugs, but also in the clinical-psychiatric research. In the psychiatric field the AMP-System proved suitable for an Electronic Data Processing (EDP) computerized data bank, which could then be applied to the processing of various scientific problems. For this reason, since 1969 all patients of the Psychiatric University Clinic of the FU Berlin are routinely recorded on this system on admission to the clinic. Similarly, since 1974 all patients of the Munich clinic are described on the AMP sheets and scales 1–4, and on discharge on AMP sheets 3 and 4. Since the introduction of the revised form of the latter sheets in January 1981, the findings at discharge are now also recorded for patients of the Berlin clinic. Consequently, the AMP (since 1978/79 the AMDP [*Guy and Ban,* 1982]) data have been the base of reference for all scientific studies involving patients in the Berlin and Munich clinics.

Which scientific queries about tests of drugs can be processed with the aid of the AMP documentation can be shown in a few examples. *Vogel* [1975] used the AMP-System to investigate the question which factors from the life history of a mentally ill person influence the course of his illness. The aim was to discover how often brain damage from early childhood occurs in a defined psychiatric population, their distribution amongst various diagnostic groups as well as the influence on the manifestation age and the course of the mental illness. Aided by an extraction program (Fortran), those with such traits, and for whom the item brain damage from early childhood was recorded 'certain' or 'questionable', were compared to a control group. In this way, out of 1,926 patients from the Psychiatric Clinic Berlin 82 patients could be found with brain damage in early childhood recorded on the AMP sheet 2 and – an essential factor – compared respectively to matched patients from the total population as a control according to age, sex and diagnosis. This showed that patients with brain damage from early childhood became ill already at a younger age than patients without this additional damage. Such an investigation with a random psychiatric population could not have been carried out had the data not been stored by EDP and were therefore recallable at any time.

The AMP-System can also be used for the recording of long-term catamnesis. For example, for over 15 years at the Berlin University Clinic patients on a long-term prophylactic lithium treatment are examined every 6 weeks and the finding is recorded on the AMP [*Müller-Oerlinghausen,* 1977]. In a catamnestic study of schizophrenic patients under long-term neuroleptic therapy, which has been carried out continuously since 1957, the AMP-System is similarly used for the documentation of the course of the illness [*Pietzcker* et al., 1981].

Besides its significance for scientific studies, the AMP-System has proved its value as one of the important instruments in the further education of candidates specializing in the field of psychopathology. It is also used in educating medical and psychology students. In using the AMP-System as a didactic instrument, it is possible to show in television films all symptoms of the classic descriptive psychopathology and to discuss these on the basis of the definition in the AMP manual.

A good training in psychopathology can be quickly achieved, since the student filling out the AMP documentation form must consider the four stages of decision, as illustrated in figure 1, and must justify his decisions in the subsequent discussion as to why he marked a particular symptom or not.

Outlook

In the revised version of 1979 as AMDP, the AMP-System has achieved an increasingly strong resonance in German-speaking areas and hopefully its sphere of application will become considerably larger. In pursuit of this hope, it was decided to compose the monograph and publish it in the English language. Having revised the system in 1979 it can be assumed that for at least another 10 years no further revision of the AMDP-System will occur. However, this does not mean that no more developments of the AMDP-System are to be expected in the near future. Further studies should enable an easier application of the AMDP-System. The formation of subscales is already being finished (*Pietzcker* et al., 1983). Until now the psychopathological symptoms have been the object of observation for the 'psychic finding' sheet, therefore called sheet 'psychopathological symptoms'. But now methods and documentation scales are being processed to comprehend the healthy parts of the personality (i.e. for the ability and competence of the patient). A group has been formed to develop a documentation instrument for this field, as well as a detailed documentation for neurotic disorders. Finally, in order to unify the collection of data, a semi-structured interview is planned by the German AMDP group.

References

Angst, J.; Battegay, R.; Bente, D.; Berner, P.; Broeren, W.; Cornu, F.; Dick, P.; Engelmeier, M. P.; Heimann, H.; Heinrich, K.; Helmchen, H.; Hippius, H.; Pöldinger, H.; Schmidlin, P.; Schmitt, W.; Weis, P.: Das Dokumentations-System der Arbeitsgemeinschaft für Methodik und Dokumentation in der Psychiatrie (AMP). Arzneimittel-Forsch. *19:* 399–405 (1969).

Angst, J.; Battegay, R.; Bente, D.; Cornu, F.; Dick, P.; Engelmeier, M. P.; Heimann, H.; Heinrich, K.; Hippius, H.; Pöldinger, W.; Schmidlin, P.; Schmitt, W.; Weis, P.: Über das gemeinsame Vorgehen einer deutschen und schweizerischen Arbeitsgruppe auf dem Gebiet der psychiatrischen Dokumentation. Schweizer Arch. Neurol. Neurochir. Psychiat. *100:* 207–211 (1967).

Angst, J.; Battegay, R.; Pöldinger, W.: Zur Methodik der statistischen Bearbeitung des Therapieverlaufes depressiver Krankheitsbilder. Methodik Inform. Med. *3:* 54–65 (1964).

Bente, D.; Engelmeier, M. P.; Heinrich, K.; Hippius, H.; Schmitt, W.: Zur Dokumentation medikamentöser Wirkungen bei der psychiatrischen Pharmakotherapie. Arzneimittel-Forsch. *11:* 886–890 (1961).

Busch, M.; Fähndrich, E.; Freudenthal, K.; Renfordt, E.: Zur Anwendung und Weiterentwicklung des AMP-Systems. Bericht über ein Symposium und Trainingsseminar. Pharmakopsychiatrie *8:* 170–175 (1975).

Cranach, M. von; Strauss, A.: Zur Weiterentwicklung des AMP-Systems. Bericht über das 2. AMP-Symposium und Trainingsseminar. Pharmakopsychiatrie *10:* 254–261 (1977).

Gebhardt, R.; Helmchen, H.: Zur Zuverlässigkeit psychopathologischer Symptomerfassung. Die Übereinstimmung mehrerer Beurteiler im AMP-System. Schweizer Arch. Neurol. Neurochir. Psychiat. *112:* 459–469 (1973).

Guy, W.; Ban, T. A.: The AMDP-system (Springer, Berlin 1982).

Heimann, H.; Angst, J.; Bente, D.; Berner, P.; Helmchen, H.; Hippius, H.: Erfahrungen der Arbeitsgemeinschaft für Methodik und Dokumentation in der Psychiatrie (AMP); in Bochnik, Pittrich, Multifaktorielle Probleme in der Medizin (Akademische Verlagsgesellschaft, Wiesbaden 1976).

Müller-Oerlinghausen, B.: 10 Jahre Lithium-Katamnese. Nervenarzt *48:* 483–493 (1977).

Pietzcker, A.; Poppenberg, A.; Schley, J.; Müller-Oerlinghausen, B.: Outcome and risks of long-term treatment with an oral neuroleptic drug. Arch. Psychiat. NervKrankh. *229:* 315–329 (1981).

Pietzcker, A.; Gebhardt, R.; Strauss, A.; Stöckerl, M.; Langer, C.; Freudenthal, K.: The syndrome scales in the AMDP-system. Mod. Probl. Pharmacopsychiat., vol. 20, pp. 88–99 (Karger, Basel 1983).

Pöldinger, W.: Über Notwendigkeit und Möglichkeiten standardisierter Befunderhebungen in der Psychiatrie; in Kranz, Heinrich, Psychiatrie im Übergang (Thieme, Stuttgart 1969).

Scharfetter, C.: Das AMP-System. Manual zur Dokumentation psychiatrischer Befunde (Springer, Berlin 1971).

Vogel, H. P.: Der Einfluss frühkindlicher Hirnschäden auf Art und Verlauf psychiatrischer Erkrankungen bei Erwachsenen. Arch. Psychiat. NervKrankh. *220:* 361–371 (1975).

Dr. E. Fähndrich, Psychiatrische Klinik und Poliklinik der Freien Universität, Eschenallee 3, D-1000 Berlin 19

Mod. Probl. Pharmacopsychiat., vol. 20, pp. 10–18 (Karger, Basel 1983)

From AMP to AMDP

E. Fähndrich, H. Helmchen
Department of Psychiatry, Free University of Berlin, Berlin, FRG

Objectives

At the Berlin Association for Methodology and Documentation in Psychiatry (AMP) Symposium in 1974 the participants agreed to undertake a first revision of the AMP-System. This decision was based on discussions in connection with joint ratings of seven video films of psychiatric patients. The aim of such a revision would be to eliminate so-called 'pool items', e.g. 'delirious', and to achieve more accurate definitions for the individual items in the manual. Moreover, an attempt was made to operationalize the social data. Further aims for future work were to intensify the AMP psychopathology training in all the participating clinics as well as an improvement of the electronic data processing (EDP).

Originally, it was intended that the AMP item documentation should remain unchanged and a comprehensive revision of the whole system was not considered, simply an improvement of the manual. This work was taken over by the working groups 'Social Data and Anamnesis', 'Psychic Findings: Glossary' and 'Somatic Findings' [1, 7]. Besides this, a further group 'Interrater Reliability' should examine the manual submitted to them in its new form by the above-named groups. It was the job of an EDP group to develop new possibilities for processing the data documented by the AMP-System. In the following, the work of one of these groups is presented as an example.

The working group 'Psychopathological Symptoms: Glossary' worked through the glossary item by item, in accordance with the assignment, and tried to improve the definitions with respect to the following objectives: (a) more precise formulation of the glossary text; (b) more distinct delimitation between the items; (c) better differentiation between items of the so-called experiential and the behavioral levels; (d) attempt to operationalize the levels of intensity-questionable, mild, moderate, severe; (e) description of the phenomena without diagnostic-nosological references, since each item was supposed to be considered by itself, independent of diagnoses.

Procedure

Before the work began all the AMP members were asked to criticize the existing system and to contribute suggestions for improvement; 125 suggestions for improvement were received for the areas of AMP sheets 3 and 4 (psychopathological symptoms and somatic signs). Here it already became clear that many were also in favor of a change in the documentation sheets. In addition to the AMP members' requests for change, several investigations [2–4] showed that not only a reformulation of the glossary for each single item according to the above-mentioned objectives but also a revision of the entire item pool of the documentation system would be necessary in order to attain a genuine improvement. On the basis of 2,613 AMP sheets for 'psychopathological symptoms' the authors had classified all of the AMP items into 'non-specific frequent – non-specific seldom, specific frequent – specific seldom'. According to this, 68 of the 123 AMP items on sheet 3 ('psychopathological symptoms') were both non-specific and seldom [4]. Based upon these investigations and the AMP members' suggestions for improvement an 'interim solution' for an AMP sheet 'psychopathological symptoms' with 115 items was drawn up. The deletion of items was, for the most part, due to these investigations; the new insertions were based more upon the requests of the AMP members. Besides this change of the item pool a new glossary with reformulated definitions of all of these items was submitted. This 'interim version' was available in 1976. In order to examine its quality, a multicenter study of interrater reliability was performed [5]; 102 raters from seven psychiatric clinics in Switzerland and Germany participated in it. They were shown 12 different videotapes, the psychopathology of which was documented on the aforesaid sheet 3 'psychopathological symptoms' according to the definitions of the temporary glossary. The results of this study of interrater reliability [5] as well as the feedback of all of the AMP members, who had likewise worked with this interim version for approximately 1 year, served as the basis for the preparation of a 'final version', which again differed considerably from the interim version. This version was accepted by the members at the AMP Symposium in Vienna in 1978 and a final commission which convened in the same year in Berlin was assigned the edition of the sheets and the manual. The revised documentation system with five sheets and an accompanying manual was published in 1979. Since that time it has no longer been called AMP but instead AMDP-System [1]. The reasons for the expansion of the abbreviation were, for one, the frequent confusion in the literature with the cyclic AMP and other organizations with the same abbreviation, a problem which had become more significant considering the international dissemination of the system. However, this was meant, above all, to express that the new version of the documentation system represented the result of an intensive, essential revision over a period of several years and thus clearly differed from the preceding version. In the following the differences between the first version (AMP-System) and the improved form (AMDP-System) are to be presented in detail.

General Changes from AMP to AMDP

(a) The two punch sheets of the AMP-System, which should serve in assessing the course of the medication at the end of treatment, were never used and were therefore no longer included in the revised AMDP version. (b) The revised AMDP-System has five documentation sheets: three serve to document the history and social data (AMDP sheets 1–3); two sheets for documenting psychopathological symptoms and autonomic-somatic-neurological abnormalities (AMDP sheets 4 and 5). (c) The items were numbered in order to increase clarity. (d) The framework of collecting data in the area of anamnesis and social data was expanded considerably. (e) The number of items in the area of psychopathological symptoms and somatic signs was reduced from 184 to 140. (f) The categories 'not estimable, because not accessible' and 'presence questionable', which were present in the old AMP-System, were combined in 'not ascertained' in the new AMDP-System. The decisional levels of 'estimability or accessibility' and 'certainty of decision' about the presence or absence of an item [fig. 1, page 5] are thereby combined in the coding 'not ascertained', which must ultimately also be marked when, contrary to the rule, one failed to examine an item. (g) So-called reserve items were introduced. These allow each working group to portray additionally those items not contained in the documentation system which it judges to be important. (h) The manual was thoroughly revised: details below.

Comparison between the AMP and the AMDP

Documentation Sheets for Case History and History of Illness (AMP sheets 1 and 2 versus AMDP sheets 1, 2, and 3)

The AMDP sheet 2 is new; it was adopted to facilitate a representing of the patient's biography in a form that is as differentiated as possible. On the basis of the 'life events' concept [6], influences are documented which in the opinion of the psychiatrist or of the patient are related to the manifestation of the illness. Moreover, a clear synoptical table of the patient's life course was developed in order to make it feasible to relate objective events to various phases of the patient's life. Newly introduced was the documentation of the duration of the rater's clinical psychiatric experience.

Documentation Sheet 'Psychopathological Symptoms' (AMP sheet 3 versus AMDP sheet 4)

The heading of this sheet was changed only slightly. Now it is possible to mark a patient's numbered position within a particular investigation or project. The assessment period can be stated in days. Finally, evidence concerning possible intelligence disturbances (estimated by the rater) are now to be marked. Due to the changes in the range of the items, some of the individual headings of item groups changed to such an extent that they took on a different meaning and for this reason had to be given new names (table I).

The number of items was reduced from 123 to 100; 82 items of the old AMP sheet 3 were contained in the revised AMDP sheet 4, 18 items were added. In all categories with the exception of 'delusion', the item 'other' was deleted because it was non-specific. A dotted line was introduced in the category 'delusion' separating those items which are necessary for the formal description from those which characterize the delusional content. The line is meant to remind the rater that two markings are required here, one for the formal description (above the line) and one for the thematic description (below the line). The items 101–115 were in-

Table I

AMP categories		AMDP categories
Obsessive ideas, compulsions, phobias	→	Phobias and compulsions
Disorders of ego and personality	→	Disorders of ego
Affective changes, disorders of feeling	→	Disturbances of affect
Disorders of psychomotility	→	Disorders of drive and motility
Dispositional abnormalities	→	Circadian disturbances
Disorders of drive and social behavior, needing nursing care	→	Other symptoms

troduced as write-in or reserve items (R items). They allow the additional documentation of special items without altering the basic pool. Moreover, there is now a general statement by the rater about the 'certainty' regarding the findings that were made.

Changes in the Individual Categories

Disorders of Consciousness. The AMP items 'delirious' and 'twilight state' were eliminated; 'lowered consciousness' (item No. 1), 'narrowed consciousness' (item No. 3) and 'expanded consciousness' (item No. 4) were introduced.

Disorders of Orientation. No changes were made here.

Disturbances of Attention and Memory. The new AMDP item 'paramnesias' (item No. 14) had previously been represented in AMP under 'other'. Otherwise, there were no changes in this area.

Formal Disorders of Thought. The AMDP item 'rumination' (item No. 20) is new. Here, the non-compulsive, constant thought absorption with a particular object is meant. This symptom could not be represented in the old AMP System.

Phobias and Compulsions. Here 'suspiciousness' (item No. 27) was added in AMDP. The non-delusional distrustful basic attitude of a person or a particularly pronounced jealousness is meant by this.

Delusions. The former AMP item 'sudden delusional ideas/delusional thoughts' was divided into two AMDP items (item No. 35 and 36). No changes were made other than slight rearrangements of the individual items.

Disorders of Perception. No changes.

Disorders of Ego. The AMP item 'Autism' was deleted. It is not a single item but rather a syndrome, which can be portrayed through the combination of individual AMDP items. The AMP item 'disorder of ego-identity' and 'other depersonalization experiences' were renamed 'depersonalization' (AMPD item No. 54) and 'derealization' (AMDP item No. 50). Along with those items already included previously, a more precise description of ego disorders now became possible.

Disturbances of Affect. Here nothing was changed in the scope of the items. The items were rearranged and occasionally renamed or changed slightly in their definitions, for example, AMDP item No. 61 'blunted affect', which in the old AMP-System was called 'impoverishment of feeling/blunted affect'. Now the apathy, indifference and 'nonchalance' of a patient is meant by this and no longer the 'moral insanity' of the old psychiatry which the item formerly emphasized.

Disorders of Drive and Motility. The AMP item 'disintegration of speech/neologisms' was eliminated, since it had been inappropriately placed under this heading. Now 'neologisms' appear as AMDP item No. 26 under the heading 'Formal disorders of thought'. The AMP items 'stupor' and 'negativism' were eliminated. 'Stupor' can now be coded under 'lack of drive' (AMDP item No. 80) as its highest degree of severity. 'Negativism' was deleted due to very low interrater reliability [5]. Special forms of negativism can be coded elsewhere, e.g. now it is possible to code negativistic speech behavior under 'mutism' (AMDP item No. 87). The item 'histrionic' was added (AMDP item No. 86); here, above all, exaggerated, stylized behavior is to be represented.

Circadian Disturbances. The AMP items 'better in a.m.' and 'exacerbation at night' were dropped because they were non-specific, seldom. For a more precise description of circadian features the items 'worse in a.m.' (item No. 89) and 'worse in p.m.' (item No. 90) were added in AMDP.

Other Symptoms. The AMP items 'feeling of being ill', 'deviation of sexual drive', 'decreased libido', 'refusal of food' and 'activities more difficult' were deleted. They were all non-specific [4]. The former AMP items 'suicidal tendencies' and 'suicidal acts' were combined under 'suicide' (ADMP item No. 95) and AMP items 'aggressive tendencies' and 'aggressive acts' to 'aggressiveness' (AMDP item No. 94); AMP item 'not able to feed self alone', 'unable to care for bodily needs', 'incontinent' and 'remains in bed' were combined to form the AMDP item 'lack of self-care' (item No. 100). AMP item 'decrease in contacts' was renamed 'social withdrawal' (AMDP item No. 92) and AMP item 'increase in contacts' changed to 'excessive social contact' (AMDP item No. 93). 'Decreased libido' is now documented as 'decreased sexual appetite' (item No. 109) on AMDP sheet 5.

Documentation Sheet 'Somatic Signs'
(AMP sheet 4 versus AMDP sheet 5)

Whereas the scale 'somatic signs' originally served, above all, to document side effects of the treatment with psychotropic drugs, its present emphasis has been shifted. Now the symptoms observable in the autonomic and somatic areas during psychiatrically relevant illnesses are supposed to be represented. For this reason, the AMDP sheets 4 and 5 are conceived of as a unit, which is expressed among other things by the consecutive numbering of the individual items.

Considerable changes were necessary due to the new concept. The headings 'other physical symptoms', 'constitutional type' and 'additional examination' of the old AMP sheet 4 were deleted. The number of items was reduced from 61 to 40; 5 new items were added. Here R items were also introduced for the aforesaid reasons.

Changes in the Individual Categories

Sleep/Vigilance Disturbances. AMP items 'tendency to fall asleep during the day' and 'increased dream activity' were deleted. 'Early wakening' (AMDP item No. 104) was included as an axial symptom of endogenous depression.

Appetite Disturbances. The item 'decreased libido' (AMDP item No. 109) was moved here. It had previously been located on the AMP sheet 3 'psychopathological symptoms'. The old AMP heading 'autonomic disturbances' was subdivided into four new AMDP headings: (1) gastrointestinal disturbances; (2) cardio-respiratory disturbances; (3) other autonomic disturbances, and (4) other somatic disturbances.

Gastrointestinal Disturbances. The item 'gastric discomfort' (AMDP item No. 114) is new.

Cardiac-Respiratory Disturbances. The former AMP item 'cardiac sensations' was subdivided into 'palpitations' (AMDP item No. 119) and 'cardiac pain' (AMDP item No. 120).

Autonomic Disturbances. The five autonomic symptoms (AMDP items No. 121–125) listed here were also present in the old AMP Scale.

Other Somatic Disturbances. 'Backache' (No. 127), 'heaviness in legs' (No. 128) and 'conversion symptoms' (No. 131) were added in the AMDP.

Neurological Disturbances. AMP items 'persisting hyperkinesis', 'paresis', 'corticospinal tract reflexes' and 'primitive reflexes' were deleted. 'Heightened muscular tone' is now called 'hypertonia' (AMDP item No. 132). The AMDP item 'tremor' (No. 134) is the combination of the former AMP items 'mild tremor' and 'moderate to severe tremor'. Moreover, the AMP information 'thorough neurological examination – yes – no' was deleted in the AMDP for didactic reasons because, if an examination is completed at all, it is always supposed to be thorough.

References

1 Arbeitsgemeinschaft für Methodik und Dokumentation in der Psychiatrie: Das AMDP-System. Manual zur Dokumentation psychiatrischer Befunde. 4. korr. u. erw. Aufl. (Springer, Berlin 1981).

2 Baumann, U.: Diagnostische Differenzierungsfähigkeit von Psychopathologie-Skalen. Arch. Psychiat. NervKrankh. *219:* 89–103 (1974).

3 Baumann, U.; Angst, J.: AMP-System: Verlaufsanalysen psychopathologischer und somatischer Symptome. Arch. Psychiat. NervKrankh. *223:* 227–238 (1977).

4 Baumann, U.; Schneidewind, G.; Angst, J.; Helmchen, H.; Hippius, H.: Untersuchungen zum AMP-System. Arzneimittel-Forsch. *26:* 1111–1114 (1976).

5 Busch, H.; Cranach, M. v.; Gulbinat, W.; Renfordt, E.; Tegeler, J.: Reliability of the AMDP-System. A preliminary report on a multicentre exercise on the reliability of psychopathological assessments. Acta psychiat. scand. *62:* 382–392 (1980).

6 Dressler, D. M.; Donovan, J. M.; Geller, R. A.: Life stress and emotional crisis: the idiosyncratic interpretation of life events. Compreh. Psychiat. *17:* 549–558 (1976).

7 Fähndrich, E.; Helmchen, H.; Hippius, H.: History of the AMDP-system. Mod. Probl. Pharmacopsychiat., vol. 20, pp. 161–173 (Karger, Basel 1983).

Dr. E. Fähndrich, Psychiatrische Klinik und Poliklinik der Freien Universität, Eschenallee 3, D-1000 Berlin 19

Mod. Probl. Pharmacopsychiat., vol. 20, pp. 19–34 (Karger, Basel 1983)

Foreign Adaptations of the AMDP-System

D. Bobon

Department of Psychiatry, University of Liège Medical School, Liège, Belgium

The development of the AMDP-System by a multicentre and supranational group of German, Swiss and later Austrian psychiatrists is reported in detail by *Fähndrich,* et al. [this volume]. The decision by five German psychiatric university departments to elaborate a collaborative rating scale for the evaluation of the antipsychotic effects of neuroleptics was taken during the 1st Nürnberger Symposium of the 'Arbeitsgemeinschaft für Neuropsychopharmakologie und Pharmakopsychiatrie' (AGNP) in 1960, as *Bente* et al. [1960, 1966] recalled. The merging of the German and Swiss efforts was decided in 1965, and anamnestic items complemented the psychopathological and somatic scales; the common standardized system was made public at the 5th congress of the Collegium Internationale Neuro-Psychopharmacologicum or CINP in Washington in 1966 [*Angst* et al., 1967]. This system was given the name AMP on the occasion of the 6th CINP congress in Tarragona in 1968 [*Angst* et al., 1969].

A Workshop on Translations of the AMP-System was held during the 10th CINP Congress in Quebec in July 1976. This was the first survey of the ongoing adaptations of the second German edition [*Scharfetter,* 1972], namely the Croatian [*Bohacek,* 1978], English [*Ban,* 1978], French [*Bobon,* 1978d], Russian [*Saarma and Morozov,* 1978] and Spanish [*Heinze,* 1978].

The rapidly increasing number of translators and foreign users of the AMP-System was also increasing the danger of a loss of the formal comparability between translations and of the conceptual identity of the symptoms measured. There was also a growing need for information on the German publications and ongoing revision efforts, and for a coordination between potential translators in a specific language. These are the reasons why *Bobon* was invited to join as International Secretary the AMP Committee which was set up on the occasion of the 50th anniversary of *Kraepelin's* death, celebrated in Munich in 1976. Since then, the *International Secretariat* in Liège acts as a coordinator between the German group and the foreign groups. It has established a communication network (Newsletters, Workshop on Translations of the AMDP-System), has assembled an updated computerized AMDP bibliography, and has organized meetings for the various groups.

An informal meeting of AMP translators was held in Honolulu in 1977 on the occasion of the VIth World Congress of Psychiatry. A 2nd Workshop on Translations of the AMP-System was included in the program of the 11th CINP Congress in Vienna in 1978 but was not published. Three new ongoing adaptations were reported at this session, namely the Greek *(Stefanis),* the Japanese *(Itoh)* and the Portugese *(Paes de Sousa).* A 3rd Workshop will be held during the VIIth World Congress of Psychiatry, again in Vienna, in 1983.

Croatian Adaptation

As claimed by *Bohacek* [1978], this was the first *complete* translation of the AMP-System, including a draft of the manual. The author did it during a stay at the Psychiatric Department of the Free University of Berlin in 1968; he has not adapted it to the 1979 revision yet.

French Adaptation

The first presentation of the pioneering efforts of five German psychiatric departments towards a standardized assessment of change under neuroleptic drugs was actually made in Berlin in 1960 during a French-German meeting on psychopharmacology [*Bente* et al., 1962].

The five Swiss university departments of psychiatry, including two French-speaking ones (Geneva and Lausanne), had developed a psychopathological and somatic scale for antidepressants. This pre-AMP scale was translated into French and applied to drug trials [*Pöldinger* et al., 1966]. The difficulties in translating its concepts were reported at the IVth World Congress of Psychiatry in Madrid in 1966 [*Dick* et al., 1968];

the translation itself was presented at the Tarragona CINP congress two years later [*Angst* et al., 1969]. But the lack of the corresponding manual and the lack of interest at that time among French-speaking psychiatrists for quantitative psychopathology hampered the success of this translation. Another adaptation of the AMP Scales in French had been done in our department in 1973; preliminary applications of this adaptation gave indications on its sensitivity [*J. Bobon* et al., 1974, 1977; *Bobon,* 1978c].

On the occasion of the 9th CINP Congress in Paris in 1974, *Dick* and *Heimann* accepted *Bobon's* proposal to revive the French adaptation of the AMP Scales by extending the core of translators to a French psychiatrist (*Dufour,* from Marseille, interested in the AMP-System since a stay at the Department of Psychiatry in Berlin), to Germans (*Mombour* and *Piree,* from the Max-Planck-Institute for Psychiatry in Munich, knowledgeable in the AMP, in French and in French psychiatry) and to a French-speaking Belgian (*Bobon,* familiar with the AMP-System since a stay at the Max-Planck-Institute for Psychiatry).

The first session of this purposely small group took place in Liège in 1975. In 8 years, it held 16 international meetings in Clermont-Ferrand, Geneva, Liège, Luxemburg, Marseille, Montreal, Munich, Quebec, Tübingen and Vienna. The number of participants steadily increased from 10 to almost 100, the range of nationalities expanding from 6 to 11 (Austria, Belgium, Canada, France, Germany, Greece, Italy, Luxemburg, Portugal, Spain and Switzerland) plus occasional representatives from Algeria and Zaïre. In a letter to an EEC Director General in March 1982, *Pichot,* President of the World Psychiatric Association, spoke of 'a remarkable effort toward international collaboration, all the more as it has been completely benevolent'.

The first edition of the French manual [*Bobon,* 1978a] was considered as a sort of 'zero edition' aimed at collecting empirical data on the difficulties encountered by French-speaking psychiatrists in applying German concepts in their AMDP quantification. This edition included both psychopathological and somatic rating scales at an intermediate stage between the 1972 German edition and its 1979 revision. It did not comprise the anamnestic parts. Its final draft had been approved during the 8th international meeting of the French-speaking section in Liège in November 1977, the first major symposium of this section ('from Iran to Quebec') on which occasion the French-Speaking Secretariat was established in Liège. The first edition of the French manual made the new initials AMDP public for the first time. It was symbolically released on the

	Absent	Léger	Moyen	Fort	Très fort	Sans avis
	0	1	2	3	4	?
1 Troubles de la concentration (10)						
2 Pensée inhibée (15)						
3 Pensée ralentie (16)						
4 Pensée appauvrie (18)						
5 Ruminations (20)						
6 Anesthésie affective éprouvée (60)						
7 Troubles de l'éprouvé vital (62)						
8 Tristesse (63)						
9 Perte d'espoir (64)						
10 Anxiété psychique éprouvée (65)						
11 Sentiment d'insuffisance (71)						
12 Sentiment de culpabilité (73)						
13 Diminution de l'énergie (80)						
14 Inhibition de l'énergie (81)						
15 Sociabilité diminuée (92)						
16 Tendances suicidaires (95)						
17 Difficultés d'endormissement (101)						
18 Réveils nocturnes (102)						
19 Réveil matinal (104)						
20 Appétit diminué (106)						
21 Fuite des idées (22)						
22 Euphorie (66)						
23 Surestimation de soi (72)						
24 Augmentation de l'énergie (82)						
25 Logorrhée (88)						
26 Sociabilité excessive (93)						
27 Absence du sentiment d'être malade (97)						

Les numéros entre parenthèses correspondent aux numéros d'items de la deuxième édition francaise (1981).

Fig. 1. Adaptation of the Zürich Mania-Depression Subscale in French [*Bobon*, 1981].

occasion of the 76th Annual Congress of the French-Speaking Psychiatrists and Neurologists, held in Charleroi in 1978 under the presidency of the heads of the Belgian and French psychiatric departments that promoted the AMDP-System in their respective country, namely, the psychopharmacologists *Jean Bobon* (Liège) and *Sutter* (Marseille).

	Absent	Léger	Moyen	Fort	Très fort	Sans avis
	0	1	2	3	4	?
1 Obsessions-phobies						
2 Hypocondrie						
3 Majoration des affects						
4 Anxiété						
5 Dépression						
6 Ralentissement						
7 Agitation, hyperactivité						
8 Humeur maniaque						
9 Tension – Irritabilité – Agressivité						
10 Délire						
11 Hallucinations-tr. d'identité-syndr. influence						
12 Discordance						
13 Tr. de conscience – Orientation – Mémoire						

Fig. 2. AMDP Syndromic Scale.

The French revision of the AMDP-System is fully compatible with the German revision. It was published on the occasion of the 15th International French-Speaking AMDP Meeting, in Montreal in 1981 [*Bobon,* 1981). A multicentre Franco-Belgian rating of 388 patients was reported at the 16th International Meeting of this section, held in Liège in 1982 in dedication to *Jean Bobon* on the occasion of his 70th anniversary and retirement. This representative sample [*Bobon* et al., 1982] (at least 25 patients from each of the following university departments of psychiatry: Brussels, Charleroi, Liège, Luxemburg, Nice, St-Etienne and Ste-Ode) demonstrates a) the great similarity between the factor structure of the AMDP Scales in French-speaking and German-speaking patients; b) the usefulness of French write-in items on anxiety in building an anxiety factor; c) the stability of the Zürich *Mania-Depression Subscale* (fig. 1), which has been shown to be reliable, valid and sensitive to antidepressants [*Woggon and Dittrich,* 1979; *Bobon,* 1981]; d) the superiority of a *13-Item Syndromic Scale* derived from AMP/AMDP factors (fig. 2) over the BPRS in the global evaluation of psychopathology.

The achievements of the AMDP French section have contributed to the improvement of the instrument without altering it: (1) Modifications of the somatic scale of the second German edition, consisting in drop-

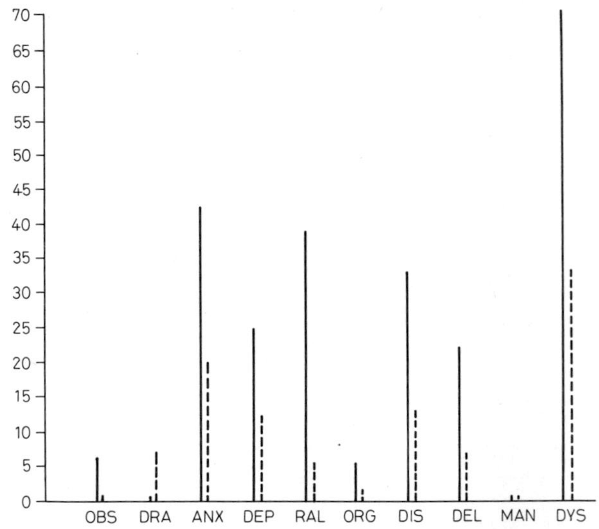

Fig. 3. Time-blind factorial profile of a delusional patient before (straight lines) and after (dotted lines) 3 weeks of a new thioxanthene, teflutixol [*Bobon and Gernay,* in prep.]. Videotaped semi-structured interview; multirater consensus item scores of the 115-item French revision of the AMDP Psychopathology Scale; factor scores (in percent) derived from the factor analysis of 388 Belgian and French patients (references in the text). OBS = Obsessions-Phobias, DRA = Dramatization, ANX = Anxiety, DEP = Depression, RAL = Retardation, ORG = Organicity, DIS = Dissociation, DEL = Delusions, MAN = Mania, DYS = Dysphoria.

ping or adding items on the basis of drug trials, systematizing the headings and introducing a standardized somatic interview; these modifications, elaborated in Liège [*Bobon,* 1978b], were first approved by the French-speaking group and then slightly modified by the German revision group; in its own revision, the French group strictly adopted this modified version; this is a typical example of a positive feedback between a foreign group and the German genitors of the system; (2) Adjunction of write-in 'reserve' items to the standard AMDP items in order to take specific needs of translators into account without altering the basic pool of German items; this innovation was also adopted by the German revision group; (3) Broadening of the range of item scores from 0–3 to 0–4 for three reasons: clinical need of two intensity levels beyond 'moderate' ('severe' and 'very severe' instead of 'severe' alone), greater a priori sensitivity to change and less central tendency. This modification was adopted in the English version but not in the German revision; (4)

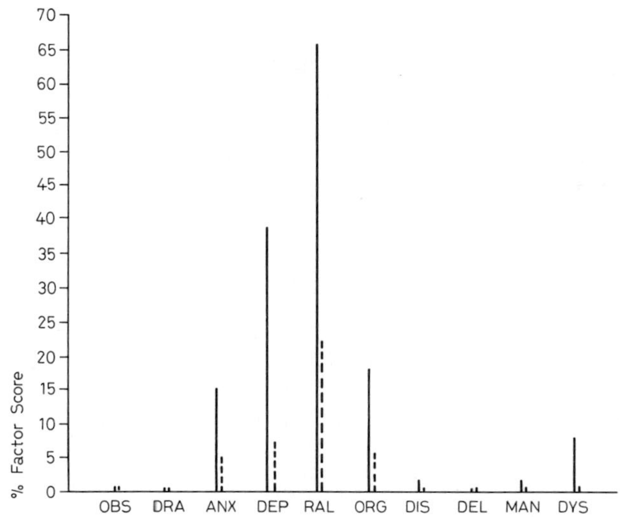

Fig. 4. Time-blind factorial profile of 5 patients before and after 3 weeks of a new antidepressant, the 5-HT blocker Ro 11-2465 (unpublished). Same methodology as fig. 3.

Elaboration of a semi-structured interview designed for the videotaped and even time-blind evaluation of the AMDP Psychopathology Scale [*Bobon* et al., 1978]; (5) Application of the scale and of the time-blind technique to drug trials: the neuroleptics bromperidol [*Bataille,* 1978] and teflutixol [*Bobon and Gernay,* in prep.], three benzamides [*Ansseau and Collard,* 1982] the tricyclic antidepressant clomipramine [*Bobon,* 1978c] and the MAO inhibitor Ro 11-1163 [*Bobon,* 1982]; figures 3 to 5 illustrate such applications in the case of the revised AMDP Psychopathology Scale; (6) Validation of the provisional Mania-Depression Scale put forward by *Woggon and Dittrich* [1979]: its depression score, in a Belgian sample, discriminates between depressed and nondepressed subjects, significantly correlates with the Hamilton Depression Scale and with the Zerssen BfS/BfS' Self-Rating Mood Scale, and is sensitive to antidepressants [*Bobon and von Frenckell,* 1980]; (7) Refinement over the years of a video methodology for the measurement of interrater reliability and eventually transcultural differences in single cases, among others by applying a modified obverse factor analysis [details in *Bobon* et al., this volume].

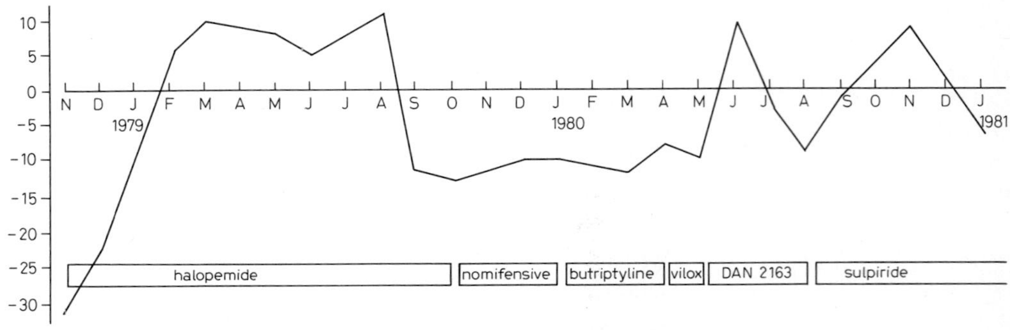

Fig. 5. Monthly evaluation over two years, with help of the French adaptation of the Zürich Mania-Depression Scale derived from the AMDP [*Woggon and Dittrich,* 1979; *Bobon,* 1981], of a bipolar depressed patient characterized by manic shifts under three different benzamides: halopemide, DAN 2163 and sulpiride [*Ansseau and Collard,* 1982].

Thanks to a number of bilingual psychiatrists who participated to the German AMDP meetings and to the French meetings as well (especially *Bobon, Mombour, Piree* and *Rein*), and thanks to the number of French-speaking departments who joined on a regular basis, terminological misunderstandings and conceptual divergences were recognized, analyzed and eliminated versus highlighted in the French manual. Let us give a few examples.

The acceptability of AMDP psychopathological terms has been increased through the exclusion of expressions defined in an idiosyncratic way in a specific department (e.g. 'interpretativeness' in the sense of delusional mood in Geneva, 'anosognosia' in the sense of lack of insight in Liège, etc).

New expressions have been coined in the case of German concepts classically ill-translated. Psychotic 'Wahnstimmung' had always been literally translated in French like in English by 'delusional mood'; the adaptators of the French manual preferred 'delusional foreboding', less literal but closer to the conceptual content of the 'Wahnstimmung'. More often, terms which had become obsolete in French psychiatry have been reintroduced in order to draw the user's attention to the unusual content of an item, e.g. 'troubles de l'aperception' for 'Auffassungsstörungen', 'pensée circonstanciée' for 'umständlich', 'perception délirante' for 'Wahnwahrnehmung'. It is noteworthy that these so-called obsolete terms are still in use in English-speaking and Spanish-speaking countries and appear in the corresponding AMDP manuals. In other words, the reappraisal of these terms in the French version has two advantages instead of one: they tend to increase the interrater reliability within French-speaking users, and they improve the terminological standardization between several translations.

The use of terminology for the improvement of interrater reliability within and between AMDP sections is also obvious if one compares the first and the second French editions [*Bobon,* 1978, 1981]. French translators had initially understood that there is only a subjective versus objective difference between inhibited and retarded thinking, hence the translation 'pensée inhibée (vécue)' versus 'pensée ralentie (observée)'; since these items refer to two qualitatively different mechanisms, the adjectives 'reported' and 'observed' have been abandoned. An opposite example concerns loss of affects. The fact that the items 'Gefühl der Gefühllosigkeit' and 'affektarm' measure the same symptom from two angles has been emphasized by the replacement of two distinct terms in the first French edition ('feeling of affective blunting', 'indifference') by 'affective anesthesia (reported)' versus 'affective anesthesia (observed)'.

All these examples are related to trivial misunderstandings due to terminology. Deeper conceptual divergences between German and French psychopathology concern delusional fabulation and drive.

Delusional fabulation or mythomania is in French psychiatry a pathognomonic symptom for paraphrenia. Now, this item has been repeatedly rejected by the Germans on the ground that it is either a formal symptom identical with a sudden delusional idea ('Wahneinfall') or a thematic symptom identical with delusions of grandeur. The following compromise has been reached between the German and the French groups: the German item 'other delusions' is, in the French manual, limited to phantastic delusions.

In their presentation of the first translation of the AMP Psychopathology Scale in French, *Dick* et al. [1968] raised the opinion that 'certain concepts, familiar in a language, seem to have no equivalent in another language. For example, the German word 'Antrieb' has no literal translation in French; more dramatic is the fact that the concept itself is absent from French psychiatry'. After numerous discussions between the German and the French AMDP groups, we came to the opposite conclusion that there is indeed a French concept corresponding to 'Antrieb', namely 'élan vital' or 'hormé', but that divergences bear on the spectrum of symptoms objectifying drive [*Bobon,* 1977, 1978 d].

In his discussion of the drive concept, *Witter* [1961] mentions a characteristic difference between French and German psychiatry: in the former one, a thorough analytic description of psychopathology is favored over a conceptual systematization, whereas in the latter one conceptualization precludes clinical subtleties. We have gained a similar impression that conceptual divergences between both might be partly due to a more global thinking among Germans against a more analytic one among Frenchmen [*Bobon,* 1977]. A typical example of such a difference concerns the German item 'depressed'. This item is the only one that has been rejected by the French adaptators of the AMDP-System on the ground that it pools a number of symptoms evaluated in several other items except for sadness. Therefore, this item is restricted to 'sadness' in the French version.

English Adaptation

The development of a translation of the AMP/AMDP-System from German to English is summarized in the 1st Workshop on Translations of the System [*Ban,* 1978] and in the introduction to the first English edition [*Guy and Ban,* 1982] and to the second French edition [*Bobon,* 1981].

Initially the psychopathological part of the second German edition of the AMP-System, namely the item list (under the name of Psychopathological Assessment Scale or PAS) and the relevant section of the manual were translated by *Saarma* in collaboration with *Ban* and *Lehmann* in Montreal. This translation was gradually improved and complemented with the anamnestic and somatic findings. In 1974, the English translation of the AMP-System was reformed by *Guy* for the Early Clinical Drug Evaluation Unit-Biometric Laboratory Information Processing System (ECDEU-BLIPS) data analysis of the NIMH. When moving to Nashville, *Ban* had to adapt this translation to US residents; in collaboration with *Jamieson,* the descriptive definitions of the items of the PAS were supplemented with operational definitions. The number of psychopathological items was inflated up to 176 and a standardized interview was developed [*Ban and Jamieson,* unpublished]. In four drug trials, the PAS compared favorably with the Brief Psychiatric Rating Scale (BPRS) and the Hamilton Rating Scale for Depression (HAMD) [*Guy and Ban,* this volume]. Another adaptation of the AMP Psychopathology Scale was also done by *Hoenig* in Newfoundland for teaching purposes but it was never published.

After the AMDP International Secretariat was created we felt that one of the major tasks of such a secretariat was to promote an official and fully compatible English adaptation of the AMDP-System based on the *Ban-Lehmann-Saarma* manuscript in collaboration with British, Canadian and US psychiatrists and psychologists on the German and French models. Preliminary contacts took place in Puerto Rico in 1979 on the occasion of the 18th Annual Meeting of the American College of Neuropsychopharmacology (ACNP). The decision to create the English-speaking section of the AMDP was taken in Edmonton in 1980 after a Workshop on the System organized by *Lapierre* within the 3rd Annual Congress of the Canadian College of Neuropsychopharmacology (CCNP). The founding meeting of this section was held in Kungälv/Göteborg on the eve of the 12th CINP Congress; during this meeting, *Ban* was asked to complete an official adaptation of the AMDP-System without delay. The final draft was approved 1 year later by an international panel of experts in German psychopathology *(J. Angst, P. Berner, D. Bobon, P. Grof, M. Hamilton, H. Helmchen, J. Hoenig, M. Hollender, R. Jamieson, E Koranyi, Y. D. Lapierre, A. Leeds, H. E. Lehmann, J. Libiger, J. Saarma* and *N. Sartorius),* in Toronto in 1981 during the 4th Congress of the CCNP. The first English edition of the AMDP-System was published in 1982 [*Guy and Ban,* 1982].

One of the major problems of the English manual was its compatibility with the French one in anticipation of its application in bilingual Canada. In this respect, the adoption by the Toronto group of several peculiarities of the French manual (especially the paper-and-pencil forms for the scales AMDP-4 and -5 as well as the 0–4 range of severity instead of the 0–3 German one) is a contribution to the uniformity of translations of the system. Other difficulties in adapting the system to Canadian psychiatry were discussed during the Quebec Workshop [*Lapierre,* 1978].

Spanish Adaptation

Independently of each other, *Heinze* in Mexico City and *J. J. López-Ibor Aliño* in Madrid translated all parts of the AMDP-System, including the glossary, into Spanish. *Heinze* based his adaptation on the second edition. He commented on it in a first paper [*Heinze,* 1976] and at the

Quebec CINP Workshop [*Heinze,* 1978]. He emphasized the difficulties in adapting socioeconomic categories such as school, occupational class or marital status.

López-Ibor Aliño adapted the 1979 German revision and swiftly published the official Spanish manual [*López-Ibor Aliño,* 1980] on the occasion of a meeting on the AMDP-System organized by him at the International Secretariat's initiative in Madrid, 1980, as a Satellite Symposium to a Regional Meeting of the World Psychiatric Association on Training Programs. An issue of the *Actas luso-españolas de Neurologia y Psiquiatria* [*López-Ibor Aliño* et al., 1982] is devoted to this symposium.

López-Ibor Aliño [1980] has also developed a microcomputer program for collecting, analyzing and retrieving all AMDP parts. This program is described in the manual and in a presentation to the Madrid symposium [*López-Ibor Aliño* et al., 1982].

One of the very first applications of the AMDP anamnestic parts comes from a Spanish psychiatrist who spent a year in Liège and noticed the potential usefulness of this part of the system [*Sanchez Blanque,* 1982].

Ongoing Adaptations

To date, we are aware of adaptations of the AMDP-System at various stages in seven other languages. The *Japanese adaptation,* worked out over several years by *Itoh* (Tokyo), has been presented at the 2nd Workshop on Translations of the AMP/AMDP-System in Vienna in 1978 [unpublished]. The complete manual is presently in press.

The *Portugese adaptation* has been made by *Paes de Sousa* (Lisbon) in close interaction with the French group. It was also presented for the first time at the Vienna CINP Workshop [unpublished]. It is now completed and should be available for the VIIth World Congress of Psychiatry in Vienna.

The *Greek adaptation* of the Psychopathology Scale and of the corresponding manual was also introduced at the Vienna Workshop, by *Stefanis* (Athens). It has been completed by *Anna Kokkevi,* his senior psychologist fluent in French, who attended several meetings of the French section in order to get an intensive training in the pitfalls of the German AMDP concepts.

Favorable results with the *Russian adaptation* of the second German edition of the AMP Psychopathology Scale were reported at the Quebec and Vienna Workshops [*Saarma and Morozov,* 1978]. The translation of the revision is under way (*Zharikov*).

The first *Italian adaptation* of the four parts of the 1972 AMP was done by *Cassano* (Pisa). A second adaptation was made by *Cazzullo and Maffei* (Milan) and was reported at the Vienna Workshop. *Cassano and Conti* are in the process of making their adaptation compatible with the English manual and with the NCDEU-BLIPS processing.

In 1982, *Bech and Kastrup* have completed a *Danish adaptation* of the AMDP Scales (in draft form).

A *Dutch adaptation* would be welcome in bilingual Belgium. It is under way at the Flemish Catholic University of Louvain *(Malfroid and Baro).*

Conclusion

Presently, there are adaptations of the AMDP-System in 11 languages, namely (a) an official Manual in English, French and Spanish; (b) a recently completed draft in Japanese and Portugese; (c) adaptations at various stages in Croatian, Danish, Dutch, Italian, Greek and Russian.

Most translations have been made on the basis of two official manuals, e.g. the German and the French or the German and the English, in order to minimize distortions of German concepts. The AMDP International Secretariat has initiated or facilitated the participation of multilingual experts in German psychopathology and/or in psychotropic drug evaluation to AMDP meetings, possibly to meetings of two distinct sections; e.g. several participants have regularly attended German and French meetings whereas others were attending French and Spanish or French and English meetings.

The difficult task of securing altogether the formal comparability of the scales, the identity of the symptoms measured and the specificity of various schools was achieved through numerous video sessions in French at which participated permanent representatives from other languages and through a number of write-in items which allow flexibility without a loss of standardization.

The international application of the AMDP-System has been handicapped until recently by the lack of an English adaptation and of short scales for frequent use in drug trials. Measurement of change has been the *Antrieb* of the AMDP group from its very beginning but it had been 'limited' on purpose by its genitors to a comprehensive evaluation of psychopathology. Drug companies have steadily supported research aimed at the development of the AMDP-System: statistical analyses, meetings, video settings, printing of manuals, secretariats, etc. Beyond the AMDP-System, they have helped setting up an international network of skilled psychopharmacologists trained in the same conceptual frame.

The AMDP Psychopathology Scale, characterized by a clear-cut distinction between the semiological and the etiopathogenetic levels as well as by the voluntary lack of criteria for determining the severity of symptoms, is particularly adequate for international research. It is not only a teaching tool and an instrument measuring change but also an instrument allowing research on the variables which influence this measurement [*Bobon* et al., this volume].

In his foreword to the English edition, *N. Sartorius,* Director of the WHO Division of Mental Health in Geneva, hails the AMDP-System as a work of outstanding value for its contribution to a common language. Says he: 'today, when multicentric collaborative studies have become a necessity and when comparative research has been recognized as a most promising research paradigm, the addition of another way to understand and compare results obtained in settings elsewhere is of tremendous importance' [*Guy and Ban,* 1982].

As stated by *Snaith* and restated by *Bech* et al. [in press] during a regional meeting of the WHO in India in 1981, time has probably arrived for a moratorium to be declared upon the publication of new scales and for researchers to spend their efforts in taking a careful look at existing scales to see how they may be improved and to compare their properties.

References

Angst, J.; Battegay, R.; Bente, D.; Cornu, F.; Dick, P.; Engelmeier, M. P.; Heimann, K.; Hippius, H.; Pöldinger, W.; Schmidlin, P.; Schmitt, W.; Weis, P.: Über das gemeinsame Vorgehen einer deutschen und schweizerischen Arbeitsgruppe auf dem Gebiet der psychiatrischen Dokumentation. Schweiz. Arch. Neurol. Neurochir. Psychiat. *100,* 207–211 (1967).

Angst, J.; Battegay, R.; Bente, D.; Berner, P.; Broeren, W.; Cornu, F.; Dick, P.; Engelmeier, M. P.; Heimann, H.; Heinrich, K.; Helmchen, H.; Hippius, H.; Lukacs, G.; Pöldinger, W.; Schmidlin, P.; Schmitt, W.; Weis, P.: Documentation clinique en psychopharmacologie: le système AMP (Arbeitsgemeinschaft für Methodik und Dokumentation in der Psychiatrie); in Cerletti, Bove. The present status of psychotropic drugs, pp. 361–365 (Excerpta Medica, Amsterdam 1969).

Ansseau, M.; Collard, J.: De la réalité du pouvoir antidépressif des benzamides: à propos d'un cas. Feuill. psychiat. Liège, *15:* 328–333 (1982).

Ban, T. A.: The AMP system in English; in Deniker et al., Neuro-psychopharmacology, pp. 1575–1579 (Pergamon Press, Oxford 1978).

Bataille, M.: Preliminary note on the antipsychotic efficacy of Bromperidol. Acta psychiat. belg. *78:* 173–179 (1978).

Bech, P.; Gastpar, M.; Morozov, P.: Clinical assessment scales for biological psychiatry to be used in WHO studies (in press).

Bente, D.; Engelmeier, M. P.; Heinrich, K.; Hippius, H.; Schmitt, W.: Methodische Gesichtspunkte zur klinischen Prüfung psychotroper Medikamente. Med. exp. *2:* 68–76 (1960).

Bente, D.; Engelmeier, M. P.; Heinrich, K.; Hippius, H.; Schmitt, W.: Projet d'une méthode de contrôle de la pharmacothérapie psychiatrique. Med. exp. *7:* suppl., pp. 11–32 (1962).

Bente, D.; Engelmeier, M. P.; Heinrich, K.; Hippius, H.; Schmitt, W.: Faktorenanalytische Untersuchungen zur Struktur psychiatrischer Merkmalszusammenhänge. Vorläufige Mitteilung. Arzneimittel-Forsch. *16:* 284–285 (1966).

Bobon, D. P.: Le concept d'Antrieb dans l'adaptation française de l'échelle psychopathologique AMP. Annls. méd.-psychol. *135:* II, 478–483 (1977).

Bobon, D. P. (ed.): Le manuel AMDP (Presses Universitaires, Liège 1978a).

Bobon, D. P.: Réflexions empiriques et bibliographiques sur l'échelle AMDP somatique. Acta psychiat. belg. *78:* 591–605 (1978b).

Bobon, D. P.: Time-blind evaluation of psychopathology in drug research. Acta psychiat. belg. *78:* 635–645 (1978c).

Bobon, D. P.: Conceptual and semantic problems raised by the French translation of the AMP Psychopathology Scale; in Deniker et al., Neuro-psychopharmacology, pp. 1583–1588 (Pergamon Press, Oxford 1978d).

Bobon, D. P. (ed.): Le système AMDP; 2e éd. (Mardaga, Bruxelles 1981).

Bobon, D. P.: La dépression: définition, mesure et classification. Revue méd. Liège, *32:* 8–13 (1982).

Bobon, D. P.; Frenckell, R. von: Rapport à la XIVe réunion AMDP francophone, non publié, Clermont-Ferrand 1980.

Bobon, D. P.; Gernay, P.: Clinical and time-blind video evaluation of the antipsychotic efficacy of teflutixol (in preparation).

Bobon, D. P.; Mormont, C.; Doumont, A.; Mirel, J.; Bonhomme, P.; Ansseau, M.; Pellet, J.; Pull, C.; De Buck, R.; Gernay, P.; Mormont, I.; Lang, F.; Lejeune, J.; Bronckart, C.: Analyse factorielle de la révision française de l'échelle AMDP. Résultats d'une étude internationale de 388 cas. Acta psychiat. belg. *82:* 371–389 (1982).

Bobon, D. P.; Mormont, C.; Mirel, J.: Un entretien psychopathologique semi-structuré adapté à l'échelle AMDP-3 et à l'évaluation vidéo en temps aveugle. Acta psychiat. belg. *78:* 606–618 (1978).

Bobon, D. P.; Mormont, C.; Mirel, J.; Fanielle, J.; Lhoist-Dericq, S.: Profil psychopathologique actuel de l'ancien prisonnier de guerre en hôpital général: intérêt de l'échelle AMP et de la vidéo; in Centre d'Etude Pour la Recherche de la Pathologie de la Captivité, pp. 107–111 (FNAPG, Bruxelles 1977).

Bobon, J.; Bobon, D. P.; Bourdouxhe, S.; Pinchard, A.: A pilot open trial of dexamisole

(R 12.563) in retarded depression. Preliminary results. J. int. med. Res. *2:* 171–174 (1974).

Bohacek, N.: First translation of the AMP system: the Croatian one; in Deniker, et al., Neuro-psychopharmacology, pp. 1565–1568 (Pergamon Press, Oxford 1978).

Dick, P.; Angst, J.; Battegay, R.; Cornu, F.; Heimann H.; Pöldinger, W.; Schmidlin, P.; Weis, P.: Problèmes des essais thérapeutiques pluricentriques (A propos d'une tentative de collaboration de 5 cliniques psychiatriques universitaires suisses); in Lopez Ibor, Proc. IVth Wld Congr. Psychiat., 2, pp. 823–825 (Excerpta Medica, Amsterdam 1968).

Guy, W.; Ban, T. A. (eds): The AMDP system (Springer, Berlin 1982).

Heinze, G.: Sistema AMP: un sistema de documentacion en psiquiatria. Psiquiat. Criminol. *6:* 36–41 (1976).

Heinze, G.: The AMP system: progress in the Spanish translation; in Deniker et al., Neuro-psychopharmacology, pp. 1571–1573 (Pergamon Press, Oxford 1978).

Lapierre, Y. D.: The implications of the AMP system in Canadian psychiatry; in Deniker et al., Neuro-psychopharmacology, pp. 1581–1582 (Pergamon Press, Oxford 1978).

López-Ibor Aliño, J. J. (ed.). El sistema AMDP (Grupo Para El Progreso de la Psiquiatria, Madrid 1980).

López-Ibor Aliño, J. J.; Rey Portolés, G.; Benitez Hita, F.; Rodriguez Gamazo, M.: Versión conversacional directa del sistema AMDP. Actas luso-esp. Neurol. Psiquiat. *10:* 429–444 (1982).

Pöldinger, W.; Angst, J.; Cornu, F.; Dick, P.; Heimann, H.: Therapeutische Erfahrungen an fünf Kliniken mit einem Dibenzoxepin-Derivat bei depressiven Zustandsbildern. Arzneimittel-Forsch. *16:* 650–653 (1966).

Saarma, J.; Morozov, G. V.: Experiences with the Russian and Esthonian translations of the AMP Psychopathology Scale in depression and schizophrenia; in Deniker et al., Neuro-psychopharmacology, pp. 1569–1570 (Pergamon Press, Oxford 1978).

Sanchez Blanque, A.: La notation des événements pathogènes en psychiatrie par le système AMDP. Différences entre malades déprimés et non déprimés. Acta psychiat. belg. *82:* 390–397 (1982).

Scharfetter, C.: Das AMP-System. Manual zur Dokumentation psychiatrischer Befunde; 2. Aufl. (Springer, Berlin 1972).

Witter, H.: 'Antrieb' als Begriff der französischen Psychiatrie. Zentbl. ges. Neurol. Psychiat. *162:* 202 (1961).

Woggon, B.; Dittrich, A.: Konstruktion übergeordneter AMP-Skalen: 'manisch-depressives' und 'schizophrenes Syndrom'. Int. Pharmacopsychiat. *14:* 325–337 (1979).

D. Bobon, M.D., Clinique psychiatrique universitaire, Rue St-Laurent 58, B-4000 Liège (Belgium)

Mod. Probl. Pharmacopsychiat., vol. 20, pp. 35–45 (Karger, Basel 1983)

AMDP Anamnestic Data: Foundations, Structure and Functions

U. Hermann

Department of Psychiatry, Free University of Berlin, Berlin

In the now authorized third version of the Association for Methodology and Documentation in Psychiatry (AMDP) system, the inventory of anamnestic characteristics was given a new design. Concerning the discussion about the causes of psychic diseases, the new form takes into account that the originally medical-biological concept is increasingly supplemented with theoretical approaches and empirical analyses which consider more sociological facts into the condition complex of psychic diseases.

Foundations of the New Concept

Historical Foundations. Already in *Comte* [14] one finds a first sociological definition of insanity as well as an investigation of the sociological qualifications for the apparition of insanity. *Comte's* [14] idea of a connection between times of social change and increasing mental disease appears in 1897 in a modified form in *Durkheim's* [24] papers on suicide. Among *Durkheim's* pupils, *Mauss* [48] contributed decisively to surmount the one-sided medical-biological concept. He was interested in the totality of the phenomenon 'human being' and he studied, for example, the effect of social stress on the psychophysical state of the individual. *Mauss'* [48] recommendation to study the human being as a total phenomenon was supplemented by *Bastide* [2] who supported multidisciplinary research, especially concerning mental diseases. The objective of a sociology of mental disorders consists – according to *Bastide* [2] – in combining the 'insanes' and those who treat them with the total field 'society', which defines simultaneously the criteria of insanity and the criteria for curing. For *Bastide* [2] the prospective patient is, from birth on, biased by familiar relations, and these familiar relations are determined by the position of this family in social class, ethnological origin, and religious confession. The social influence of the individual can also be found in the so-called psychobiologic theory of *Meyer* [50a], which says that mental disorders are to be seen as consecutive misadaptations of human beings to the physical, psychic, and social environment. Sociologic theories by *Cooley* [15] and *Mead* [49] take up the connection of psychic illness and environment insofar as they especially emphasize the importance of primary groups for the development of personality and the social process coming off it.

Considering early empirical studies concerning the research on social conditions of psychic disorders, the study by *Faris and Dunham* [30] is one of the most famous papers from the 1930s; it investigates the environmental conditions of frequent psychic illness in Chicago: on the basis of first-admitted psychically ill patients these authors were able to prove that the greatest concentration of admission rates with the diagnosis 'schizophrenia' was found downtown and the rates decreased clearly towards the suburbs. Some more social correlates of mental illness were shown in the studies preferentially carried out in capitals after World War II, e.g. the stress of town life in the Manhattan study by *Srole and Langner* [63], the corresponding to the lower social class, especially shown by *Hollingshead and Redlich* [35] in their New Haven study, the social disintegration shown by *Leighton and Hughes* [46] when investigating the underprivileged municipalities of Stirling County and the integration problem of blacks in North US capitals shown in the Philadelphia study by *Parker and Kleiner* [55].

Recent Results. One of the most consistent results in the field of psychiatric epidemiology is that persons coming from low socioeconomic classes in capitals bear a higher risk to suffer from schizophrenia. In a review of 17 studies *Eaton* [26] found in 15 that schizophrenia occurred increasingly as the social class fell. In a review of 7 international studies *Dohrenwend* [20] noted that 5 of 7 studies showed the above-mentioned inverted relation. Attempts to interpret the etiological importance of the inverted correlations between frequency of illness and appertaining class under the aspect of social causing or social selection failed mostly at the question: 'What is cause and what is consequence?'. In the analysis of 11 studies, which concern the cause-consequence relation, *Eaton and Lasry* [28] found a support of the selection, i.e. drift interpretation: in 7 studies either downward social mobility was found in schizophrenic patients or the upward social mobility was lower than expected. These results do not exclude the additional possibility of a social cause, but they show – according to *Eaton* [27, p.150] 'that schizophrenics are disabled in the modern occupational system'.

The consideration of the selection, i.e. drift hypothesis, moves along with the attention given to the importance of genetic factors in schizophrenic diseases. Among others, *Kohn* [44, 45] tried to reformulate the relationship of class, family, and schizophrenia, genetic factors, stress and conditions of living, which are bound to the socioeconomic status, and bring it in a coherent interpretation of schizophrenia. According to *Kohn* [44, 45] schizophrenia is the result of a genetically conditional potential and of a limited capability to cope with environmental stress. This hypothesis can be tested for all kinds of disorders, which raises the problem of the relative etiological relevance of social environment and heredity.

That genetic factors could be part of the etiology of psychic disorders is also shown by *Ban and Petrie* [1]. They found that the incidence rate of children having schizophrenia is ten times higher compared to the normal population when one parent is affected. If both parents are schizophrenic, the risk increases to 40%. The recent investigations of monozygotic twins and adopted children show that there exists a concordance in 47% of the cases in monozygotic twins [47]. When monozygotic twins lived apart from early childhood on, they showed a concordance concerning schizophrenia to the same extent as twins who grew up together. Furthermore, children of schizophrenics, who were adopted early, developed schizophrenic diseases at a frequency above the common illness rate of the total population. A further result which indicates the importance of genetic factors is that children of normal parents who grew up at foster parents, and of whom one parent became schizophrenic, did not show a higher schizophrenia rate [32a, 41, 42].

Although the above-mentioned studies give ground for presuming a clear hereditary influence, one must keep in mind that results in question are correlations and not well-grounded causal combinations. Therefore, one should note the positive results of adoption studies, e.g. that they do not demonstrate the respective effect of genetic and biological factors, or how schizophrenia is promoted.

Kinney and Jacobsen [43] propose to solve this problem with a differentiated comparison of the rearing environment, for example of persons with a high and low genetic risk. Critical notes to the twin research [64] show that the hitherto existing methodological problems – small samples for very complex problem constellations – must at first be overcome in order to be able to find out where the borders of environmental influence end and where the dispositional conditions exist.

A more recent medical-sociological field of research, the so-called life-event research, can help to develop and improve etiology models in psychiatry, as will be considered in the following.

The life-event approach belongs to the wider field of social etiology. It can be understood as a part of stress research as far as it localizes causal complexes for somatic or psychic diseases in biographical events, which disturb or impair the life pattern of the individual. The different trends of the life-event thinking, i.e. the studies by *Rahe* [61a] and Rahe et al. [59, 60], *Dohrenwend and Dohrenwend* [19, 21], and *Brown and Birley* [9], *Brown* et al. [11] and *Brown and Harris* [13], are distinguished primarily by their methodological approach: *Rahe* and *Dohrenwend* consider that a certain life event has an objectively corresponding pathogenic effect. The event itself *(Rahe),* or the change of the usual activities of the individual *(Dohrenwend),* are seen as decisive in this context. However, *Brown* defends the thesis that the event must be referred to the biographical constellation by which the individual is working it up. *Katschnig* [40] mentions in this connection the long-range effect of events which are past for some time and which have to a certain extent created a disposition for the development of psychic disorders, actualized when certain key events repeat themselves. *Dressler* et al. [23] and *Donovan* et al. [22] already made reflections going in the same direction; they differentiated in their general stress model between prestress life context and stress-precipitating events. *Brim and Ryff* [6, p.367] distinguished biological, social, physical and psychological events and designated their life-event concept as 'integral to the study of life-span development'.

Surveying the studies of this problem, it appears important for future research to differentiate the differing kinds of life events according to their distinct release functions, whereby the integration into the life historical context as well as the personal importance of the event to the individual should be taken likewise into account. Concerning the substantial selection of life events which should be analyzed regarding their different release functions for psychic diseases, empirical results obtained so far indicate the importance of family events such as marriage [16], death of a parent, partner, or brother/sister [4, 54], divorce or separation [5a, 7, 8], birth of children [53, 58], but also of common social events such as a move [33, 38], loss of employment [10], or professional upward/downward mobility [61a]. *Myers* et al. [52] designate this group as 'biopsychosocial events', i.e. events which have a high probability of happening during the life cycle of a human being at a certain age, but which possess releasing potential for psychic disorders only for persons with a certain grade of vulnerability. In addition to these 'biopsychosocial events', somatic events such as head injuries [17] or other somatic disorders [25, 39] are considered as life events. Furthermore, long-lasting problems can be regarded in the sense of 'events', as e.g. difficult partner relationships [36], difficult financial situation [13], quarrels with colleagues [57] or loneliness [37], which have releasing functions for illness.

Regarding the question which kinds of life events are connected with certain diagnostic categories, *Brown* et al. [11, 12] showed that life events play an important role at the start of schizophrenia and also at the start of a depression, but these authors are of the opinion that life events play the role of releasing a preexisting schizophrenia, whereas they have a direct causal effect in depression. Concerning the frequency of stress and crises before admission of schizophrenic and depressive patients, *Beck and Worthen* [3] demonstrated that 'clear triggering' could be shown in only half of the schizophrenic patients, compared with 95% of the depressive patients. Similar results were obtained by *Paykel* et al. [56], comparing depressive patients with a control group of normal persons.

Distinguishing between events which result in exits of persons and events which cause entrances of persons in the social environment of the patient, certain authors made the experience that the life events before getting depressive are mostly exit events. Trying to specify exit events in different subgroups of depression, *Brown* et al. [12] found a relation between the development of a 'neurotic depression' and the 'separation of parents during the patients' childhood', on one side, and between a 'psychotic depression' and the 'death of a parent during the childhood' on the other side.

Although these results show up trends between life events and depression and/or other psychiatric diseases, a number of studies show that in the psychiatric life-event research the dependent variable 'mental disorder' has not been treated, although problematical enough, while the independent variable 'life events' is not unequivocal and defined in detail.

Furthermore, they pointed to the fact that some additional intervening variables must be taken into account in order to explain the positive but low correlations between life-event values and psychic diseases. *Brown and Harris* [13] so showed that stressful life events especially cause depressive reactions when there are additional vulnerability factors, e.g. loss of the mother by death or separation before the age of eleven. Further intervening variables next to the above-mentioned example of a social characteristic are socioeconomical variables [18] as well as individual psychological characteristics [31].

The diversity of the cause-effect relationship in the so far delineated different concepts supports the already described trend by *Siegler and Osmond* [62] to start from a 'plurality of concepts' and no more from one single generally accepted model. In order to be able to take a decision between two contrasting concepts, the anamnestic field was conceived so that the data collection allows the verification of the different hypotheses.

Structure of the Anamnestic Documents AMDP-1 to AMDP-3

In order to be able to collect systematically the typical characteristics of the different concepts in psychiatric patients, three documentation forms were developed for the anamnestic field. The first document comprises characteristics to the clinic admission, to the school and professional education as well as to the familiar and socioeconomical total situation just before the admission. The operationalization of the professional situation, the living area, and the income area through social indicators by *Zapf* [65, 66] contribute to provide more systematic and comparability of research results and allow furthermore to relate the data obtained in a clinic area with results of sociological and psychiatric field studies.

The second anamnestic document was developed in order to get close to the present situation of the psychic ill, an also mostly multilateral image of his/her biographic total situation in connection with the life-event conception of *Dressler* et al. [23] and *Donovan* et al. [22]. On this second document it is possible to measure the environmental influences resulting in the special manifestation of illness on the present clinic admittance as seen by the patient or physician. On the other hand, a life-course schedule was elaborated in accordance to the development states of *Erikson* [29], and *Munley* [51], which serves to note the objective life changes during different developmental states of the patient as mentioned by *Rahe, Dohrenwend,* and *Brown*. In order to bring these changes of the life situation in the social area into relation with manifestations with neurotic or psychotic symptoms, with suicide attempts, addiction, or different somatic disorders, these characteristics are also measured further on the life-course schedule. The different psychosocial events as well as the different diseases were defined hereby clearly and in detail. It is possible to connect them as to kind, number, and date in the individual life course.

The third anamnestic document consists in characteristics, which are also defined in the glossary, concerning the present illness of the patient, the beginning of the disease as well as its course. Anamnestic data concerning family, suicides and suicide attempts of relatives are also included in the third document.

A first recommendation as to the design of the above-mentioned anamnesis exists since 1976. The applicability of these three forms was tested in six psychiatric hospitals; the anamnestic conception proved successful regarding its basic principles.

Functions

A main goal of the 3 anamnestic documents consists in processing detailed information to the psychic and social development of the psychic ill as well as characteristics of his/her 'illness-career', which existed so far only in the form of the case history, in order to be computerized. Therewith, the anamnestic documentation will offer possibilities to investigate correlations of social characteristics with psychic or somatic data, and aim the future goal, i.e. to elaborate foundations for a more specified life-event research.

The practicability test, which was concentrating on the methodological aspect of the measurement of anamnestic data, showed that the central life events mentioned in the second anamnestic document are in general suitable and practicable: in the column 'supposedly precipitating stress', a high rate of multiple marks was found, i.e. up to 82%. The fact that the chosen ill-making factors were not supposed by the patient nor the physician was confirmed in 20% of the cases. Changes of the life situation in a biographical context could be demonstrated and documented in 95% of the patients.

The newly elaborated anamnestic documents enable an empirical verification of kind, number, and schedule of life events (AMDP-2) in retrospective and prospective studies, i.e. its relation with the beginning of certain diseases. For such relational analyses, the first investigational step is to look for homogeneous disease groups of psychiatric patients and to check if they are marked by a specific constellation of events [34]. Homogeneous disease groups can be classified roughly by diagnosis (AMDP-3), or differentiated by psychopathologic syndromes obtained descriptively (AMDP-4). If the dependent variable 'psychic disorder' is looked at with more differentiation, as described, future secured statements will become possible as to the yet clinically orientated life-event research.

In the English and French manuals [5b, 32b], each anamnestic part has been given a specific name like the subsequent rating scales, namely *demographic data* (AMDP-1), *life events* (AMDP-2) and *psychiatric history* (AMDP-3). Giving up the frame of the opscan sheets, the adaptators of these two manuals have succeeded in replacing or adding categories within AMDP items in order to comply with regional needs, such as mother tongue.

At the XVIth International Meeting of the French-Speaking AMDP Section, in Liège in 1982, pilot applications of the anamnestic parts of the AMDP-System have been reported [61b]; these parts have been praised as the most original and potentially useful part of the system.

References

1 Ban, T.A.; Petrie, W.M.: Psychopharmacological treatment of schizophrenia. Publ. Hlth. Rev. *7:* 223–248 (1978).

2 Bastide, R.: Sociologie des maladies mentales (Flammarion, Paris 1965).

3 Beck, J.C.; Worthen, K.: Precipitating stress, crisis theory and hospitalization in schizophrenia and depression. Archs. gen. Psychiat. *26:* 123–129 (1972).

4 Birtchnell, J.: Recent parent death and mental illness. Br. J. Psychiat. *116:* 289–297 (1970).

5a Bloom, B.L.; Asher, S.J.; White, S.W.: Marital disruption as a stressor: a review and analysis. Psychol. Bull. *85:* 867–894 (1978).

5b Bobon, D.P. (éd.): Le système AMDP; 2e éd (Mardaga, Bruxelles 1981).

6 Brim, O.G.; Ryff, C.D.: On the properties of life events; in Baltes, Brim, Life-span development and behavior, vol. 3, pp. 367–388 (Academic Press, New York, 1980).

7 Briscoe, C.W.; Smith, J.B.; Robins, E.; Marten, S.; Gaskin, F.: Divorce and psychiatric disease. Archs. gen. Psychiat. *29:* 119–125 (1973).

8 Briscoe, C. W.; Smith, J. B.: Depression in bereavement and divorce. Archs. gen. Psychiat. *32:* 439–443 (1975).

9 Brown, G. W.; Birley, J. L. T.: Crisis and life changes and the onset of schizophrenia. J. Hlth soc. Behav. *9:* 203–214 (1968).

10 Brown, G. W.; Birley, J. L. T.: Social precipitants of severe psychiatric disorders; in Hare, Wing, Psychiatric epidemiology (Oxford University Press, London 1970).

11 Brown, G. W. et al.: Life-events and psychiatric disorders. 1. Some methodological issues. Psychol. Med. *3:* 74–87 (1978).

12 Brown, G. W.; Harris, T. O.; Copeland, J. R. M.: Depression and loss. Br. J. Psychiat. *130:* 1–18 (1977).

13 Brown, G. W.; Harris, T. O.: The social origins of depression (Tavistock Publications, London 1978).

14 Comte, A.: Cours de philosophie positive (von Bd. 4 ab), Discours sur l'esprit positif, 1844, Catéchisme positiviste, 1849; zit. nach Bastide, Soziologie der Geisteskrankheiten, p. 22 (Kiepenheuer & Witsch, Köln 1973).

15 Cooley, C. H.: Human nature and social order (Glencoe, New York 1902).

16 Davis, D. L.: Psychiatric illness in those engaged to be married. Br. J. prev. soc. Med. *10:* 122–127 (1956).

17 Dencker, S. J.: A follow-up study of 128 closed head injuries in twins using cotwins as controls. Acta psychiat. neurol. scand. *123:* suppl., pp. 1–125 (1958).

18 Dohrenwend, B. S.: Social status and stressful life events. J. Personal. soc. psychol. *28:* 225–235 (1973).

19 Dohrenwend, B. S.; Dohrenwend, B. P.: Stressful life events. Their nature and effects (Wiley & Sons, New York 1974).

20 Dohrenwend, B. P.: Sociocultural and social-psychological factors in the genesis of mental disorders. J. Hlth soc. Behav. *16:* 365–392 (1975).

21 Dohrenwend, B. S.; Dohrenwend, B. P.: Some issues in research on stressful life events. J. nerv. ment. Dis. *166:* 7 (1978).

22 Donovan, J. M. et al.: Psychiatric crisis. J. nerv. ment. Dis. *161:* 172 (1975).

23 Dressler, D. M.; Donovan, J. M.; Geller, R. A.: Life stress and emotional crisis: the idiosyncratic interpretation of life events. Compreh. Psychiat. *17:* 549 (1976).

24 Durkheim, E.: Le suicide; 9th ed. (Alcan, Paris 1930; English version: Glencoe, New York 1951).

25 Eastwood, M. R.; Trevelyan, M. H.: Relationship between physical and psychiatric disorder. Psychol. Med. *2:* 363–372 (1972).

26 Eaton, W. W.: Residence, social class and schizophrenia. J. Hlth soc. Behav. *15:* 289–299 (1974).

27 Eaton, W. W.: A formal theory of selection for schizophrenia. Am. J. Sociol. *86:* 149–158 (1980).

28 Eaton, W. W.; Lasry, J. C.: Mental health and occupational mobility in a group of immigrants. Soc. Sci. Med. *12:* 53–58 (1978).

29 Erikson, E. H.: Die acht Phasen des Menschen; in Erikson, E. H., Kindheit und Gesellschaft (Klett, Stuttgart 1974).

30 Faris, R. E. L.; Dunham, H. W.: Mental disorders in urban areas (Chicago Press, Chicago 1939).

31 Gorsch, R. L.; Key, M. K.: Abnormalities of pregnancy as a function of anxiety and life stress. Psychosom. Med. *36:* 352–363 (1974).

32a Gottesman, I.; Shields, J.: Rejoinder toward optimal arousal and away from original din. Schiz. Bull. *2:* 447–453 (1976).

32b Guy, W.; Ban, T. A.: The AMDP system (Springer, Berlin 1982).

33 Hall, P.: Moving house in the etiology of psychiatric symptoms. Proc. R. Soc. Med. *57:* 83–86 (1964).

34 Hermann, U.; Freudenthal, K.: Life events and psychiatric disorders (in preparation).

35 Hollingshead, A. B.; Redlich, F. C.: Social class and mental illness (Wiley, New York 1958).

36 Holmes, T. H.; Rahe, R. H.: The social readjustment rating scale. J. psychosom. Res. *11:* 213–218 (1967).

37 Ilfeld, F. W.: Characteristics of current social stressors. Psychol. Rep. *39;* 1231 (1976).

38 Jacobs, S.; Myers, J.: Recent life events and acute schizophrenic psychosis: a controlled study. J. nerv. ment. Dis. *162:* 75 (1976).

39 Karasu, T. B.; Waltzman, S. A.; Lindenmayer, J. P.; Buckley, P. J.: The medical care of patients with psychiatric illness. Hosp. Comm. Psychiat. *31:* 463–472 (1980).

40 Katschnig, H.: Sozialer Stress und psychische Erkrankung (Urban & Schwarzenberg, München 1980).

41 Kessler, S.: Progress and regress in the research on the genetics of schizophrenia. Schiz. Bull. *2:* 484–489 (1976).

42 Kety, S. S.; Rosenthal, D.; Wender, P. H.; Schulsinger, F.: Studies based on a total sample of adopted individuals and their relatives why they were necessary, what they demonstrated and failed to demonstrate. Schiz. Bull. *2:* 413–428 (1976).

43 Kinney. D. K.; Jacobsen, B.: Environmental factors in schizophrenia: New adoption study evidence and its implications for genetic and environmental research; in Wynne, Cromwell, Matthysse, The nature of schizophrenia, pp. 38–52 (Wiley & Sons, New York 1978).

44 Kohn, M. L.: Social class and schizophrenia: a critical review and formulation. Schiz. Bull. *7:* 60 (1973).

45 Kohn, M. L.: The interaction of social class and other factors in the etiology of schizophrenia. Am. J. Psychiat. *133:* 177 (1976).

46 Leighton, A.; Hughes, J.: Cultures as causation of mental disorder. Causes of mental disorder: a review of epidemiological knowledge, 1959 (Milbank Mem. Ed., New York 1961).

47 Mathysse, S. W.; Kidd, K. K.: Estimating the genetic contribution to schizophrenia. Am. J. Psychiat. *133:* 185–191 (1976).

48 Mauss, M.: Rapports réels et pratiques de la psychologie et de la sociologie. J. Psychol. normale pathol. (1924); neu gedruckt in Sociologie et Anthropologie (Presses Universitaires, Paris 1950).

49 Mead, G. H.: Mind, self and society (University of Chicago Press, Chicago 1934).

50 Meyer, A.: Psychobiology: a science of man compiled and translated by E. E. Winters and A. H. Bowers (Thomas, Springfield 1958).

51 Munley, P. H.: Erikson's theory of psychosocial development and career development, J. Vocat. Behav. *10:* 261–269 (1977).

52 Myers, J. K.; Lindenthal, J. J.; Pepper, M. P.: Life events and psychiatric impairment. J. nerv. ment. Dis. *152:* 149–157 (1971).

53 Paffenbarger, R. S.: Epidemiological aspects of parapartum mental illness. Br. J. prev. soc. med. *18:* 189–195 (1964).

54 Parkes, C. M.: Recent bereavement as a cause of mental illness. Br. J. Psychiat. *110:* 198–204 (1964).

55 Parkers, S.; Kleiner, R. J.: Mental health in an urban Negro community (Glencoe, New York 1966).

56 Paykel, E. S.; Myers, J. K.; Dievelt, M. N.; Klerman, G. L.; Lindenthal, J. J.; Pepper, M. P.: Life events and depression: a controlled study. Archs gen. Psychiat. *21:* 753–760 (1969).

57 Paykel, E. S.; Prusoff, B. A.; Myers, J. K.: Suicide attempts and recent life events: a controlled comparison. Archs gen. Psychiat. *32:* 327–333 (1975).

58 Pugh, T. F.; Jerath, B. K.; Schmidt, W. H.; Reed, R. B.: Rates of mental disease related to childbearing. New Engl. J. Med. *268:* 1224–1228 (1963).

59 Rahe, R. H. et al.: Social stress and illness onset. J. psychosom. Res. *8* (1964).

60 Rahe, R. H.; Gunderson, E. K. E.; Pugh, W. M.: Illness prediction studies. Archs envir. Hlth *25:* 192–197 (1972).

61a Rahe, R. H.: Epidemiological studies of life-change and illness. Int. J. Psychiat. Med. *6:* 133 (1975).

61b Sanchez Blanque, A.: La notation des événements pathogènes en psychiatrie par le système AMDP. Différences entre malades déprimés et non déprimés. Acta psychiat. belg. *82:* 390–397 (1982).

62 Siegler, H.; Osmond, H.: Models of madness. Br. J. Psychiat. *112:* 1193–1203 (1966).

63 Srole, L.; Langner, S.: Mental health in the metropolis: the Midtown Manhattan Study (McGraw Hill, New York 1962).

64 Woehlcke, M.: Soziologisch relevante Fragen und methodische Probleme der Zwillingsforschung. Köln, Soziol. Sozialpsychol. *29:* 319 (1977).

65 Zapf, W. (ed.): 2. Arbeitskonferenz Soziale Indikatoren. Berichte und Diskussionen (Campus, Mannheim 1974).

66 Zapf, W.: Applied social reporting: a social indicators for West Germany Society. Soc. Indicat. Res. *6:* 397–419 (1979).

Dr. Ursula Hermann, Dipl.-Soz., Department of Psychiatry, Free University of Berlin, Eschenallee 3, D-1000 Berlin 19 (West-Germany)

Mod. Probl. Pharmacopsychiat., vol. 20, pp. 46–54 (Karger, Basel 1983)

The Psychopathological Background of the AMDP-System

C. Scharfetter

Psychiatric University Hospital, Research Department, Zürich, Switzerland

The Association for Methodology and Documentation in Psychiatry (AMDP) system [1 a, b] is a derivative of the 'classical' psychopathology of the 19th and 20th century, when psychiatrists and neurologists tried to describe 'abnormal' behaviour of mental patients and to focus on 'pathognomonic' signs for categorization in syndromes or even disease entities. Modern methodological considerations stressed on an improvement of operationalization of psychopathological items, on a standardized elaboration and documentation of these data – as a common basis for empirical studies in various centres. For that purpose the founders of AMDP created out of the historically grown knowledge of psychiatry this system of standardized data sheets.

The aim of this paper is to show the problems of that psychopathology in regard of objectivity, information gathering, homo-versus heterogeneity, operationability, observer dependency, etc. In spite of the critical remarks it should not be overseen that AMDP contents a condensation of many clinicians' experiences and a progress toward a more scientific elaboration of this difficult field.

The AMDP-System Is Based on Traditional Psychopathology

The aim of this psychopathology is observation and description of 'single facts of the abnormal mental life'[7]. The prerequisite of this 'descriptive' psychopathology is the subdivision of 'abnormal' experience and behaviour into separated deviations from what is conceived as 'normal psychological functions'. This type of 'elementary' psychopathology has its own 'home-made' psychology, namely the 'elementary psychology' of *Kraepelin* [9], derived from the elementarism of *Wundt* [13].

The statement of the derivation of this descriptive psychopathology does not mean that it is itself based on one single and clear-cut demonstrable paradigm. There is by no means a strictly defined scientific basis of this traditional psychopathology which may be rather seen as a conglomerate of various and often highly individualistic condensates of the clinician's personal concept of what he calls 'abnormal' or even 'pathologic'. The approaches by authors like *Kahlbaum* [8a, b], *Hecker* [6], *Kraepelin* [9], and later by *Schneider* [11], and *Gruhle* [5] (to quote only a few names) are not closely related to *Bleuler's* [3] more interpretative (psychodynamic) view or later holistic concepts such as *Conrad's* [4] 'Gestalt-psychological concept'. In spite of these various concepts of psychopathology, a process of filtration may be seen resulting in the stressing of some basic elementary features for describing relevant experience and behaviour in psychiatry.

Objective and Subjective Information and the Interactional Dependence of Psychopathology: Experience and Behaviour

Psychopathology as an indispensable element of psychiatry – and in this sense as a practically relevant science and not only as a 'field of speculation' – has to relate not only to 'purely objectively observable' phenomena (insofar as that would be possible at all), but also to a lot of data gathered by exploring a patient on his ('inner') experience (thus sometimes helping the patient to become aware of it), and on his own functional interpretative connection ('understanding') of his experience and behaviour. Thus, psychopathology, as a branch of social science, especially has to take into consideration the 'Rosenthal effect' i.e. the influence of the observer and the situation of observation on the observable phenomena: the patient presenting symptoms and signs is not an independent object, but is determined by the social constellation of being under psychiatric observation (outdoors or indoors).

Every Observation Includes Interpretation

Even 'objective' observation and linguistically determined description includes a certain – and not well-defined – amount of interpretation deriving from (1) the patient's own personality as a result of socialization and social situation, and (2) the psychiatrist's professional approach depending on his personality, culturalization and anthropological concepts.

The Sedimentation of a Set of Psychopathological Items

In spite of the objections to the possibility of an objective, strictly empirical psychopathology, the historical development of psychiatry as a practical science has led to a set of items (psychopathological signs) useful for sharing and exchanging experience and knowledge about mental patients in daily clinical needs and in research.

Evaluation and Documentation of Psychopathological State: Self-Rating, Standardized, Semi-Standardized, and Free Interview, Item List

As questionnaires are of a very limited applicability in psychiatry, i.e. in organic and functional psychoses, rating scales for standardized or semi-standardized interviews were to be developed which led to a sufficient consensus of various observers (interrater reliability) concerning the phenomena studied for a special purpose. Content and linguistic formulation of interview questions are given, even the sequence of their presentation such as Inpatient Multidimensional Psychiatric Scale (IMPS) by *Lorr* et al. [10], and Present State Examination (PSE) *by Wing* et al. [12].

AMDP – A Symptom Checklist

The AMDP founders relied on another way of standardized documentation of their observations: they established a catalogue of psychopathological terms stemming from the traditional psychiatric experiences as laid down in monographs and textbooks of various clinicians of different schools and correspondingly with different nosological categorization.

The AMDP Focuses on 'Major' Psychopathology

Nevertheless, they agree with the gross subdivision of psychotic and non-psychotic psychiatric illnesses, the former including organic ones and the so-called functional (endogenous) psychoses (the boundaries of it varying a great deal), the latter including neurotic disturbances and personality disorders. The AMDP psychopathology is mainly concerned with the group of psychotic disorders.

The AMDP Items – A Collection of Symptoms, Syndromes, Theoretical Constructs, Personality Features, Mood Qualities, Character Traits, and Pecularities

The selection of items reflects clinical experience rather than scientific evaluation methods. Thus, the AMDP took over the traditional elements and functional groups of the older prescientific psychology and psychopathology, mixing together items of highly variable complexity, concreteness or theoretical constructions.

'Overloaded' Items

For instance: the item 'optic hallucinations' includes many different forms of visual experiences the subject does not share with others. It may occur in a clear or in a disturbed state of consciousness, in a wakeful, hypo- or hyper-aroused state, in somatically healthy or organically ill persons. It may have a biographical psychological meaning or not. It can vary between scenic visions and photomas. The weight of the concrete sign 'optic hallucinations' as a symptom depends on all these features. But all these phenomena are collected in one item.

Items Representing a Theoretical Construct

The item 'autism' (in AMP, but eliminated in AMDP) was by far not a clear and with consensus observable and definable phenomenon, but a highly complex theoretical construct, developed by *Bleuler* [3] as a basic feature of a schizophrenic person's relation to intersubjectively sharable 'reality' (autistic thinking according to *Bleuler* is dereistic conceiving). But later authors understand by 'autism' often a form of social withdrawal (in spite of the fact that an autistic person may pay more attention to the surrounding world than a non-autistic one).

Items Anticipating Diagnostic Decisions

'Autism' may serve for another important aspect concerning the item selection: it is highly determining the diagnosis – thus as an item anticipating diagnostic decisions which should rather be the result of the integration of the whole psychopathological status in cross-section, development, and course with all the other data from history and somatic state. This consideration led to the elimination of the item 'autism' in the revised AMDP.

Items Naming a Syndrome

The item 'delirious' of AMP is an example for a diagnostic syndromatic category and not a psychopathological sign constituting together with others a syndrome. Therefore, it was eliminated in the AMDP.

Item Selection from Broader Polymorphous Experiences

The item group 'ego disorders' may serve as an example for the predetermination in the item selection process. There are only few psychopathological phenomena included, not covering the broad spectrum of possible experiences of ego disorders in neurosis, depression, narcissistic and borderline conditions, and schizophrenics. The selection of items had to take into consideration which items (1) would probably be most important for diagnostic categorization, and (2) which would be the clearest definable for operationalization leading to a sufficient interrater consensus.

The Item Sample – A Collection of 'Objectively' Observable, 'Subjective' (Introspectively Detectable), and Mixed Items

About half of the items of the AMDP represent 'subjective' items (symptoms), e.g. phobia, hearing of voices, feeling of insufficiency. 'Objective' items are for example incoherent thinking, parakinesia, disorders of orientation. In some items both subjective introspective and objective information contribute to a varying degree to the decision process, e.g. disorders of concentration, delusional mood.

Psychopathological Items Are Hard to Define

The task of clear operationalization of items is not yet sufficiently solved (this could not be achieved by the new version of the AMDP either). For example the items 'inhibited thinking' and 'retarded thinking' are difficult to discern. The same is true for the items 'lack of drive' and 'inhibition of drive'.

The 'delusion' group of items includes even more hardly definable items: the definition of delusional ideation and 'delusional ideas' is not sufficiently clear. The operationalization of 'delusional mood' is insufficient, the same is true for 'systematized delusions' and even more so for 'delusional dynamics'.

Items Highly Susceptible to the Rater's Personality

The item group on mood disorders includes items the rating of which is highly dependent on the rater's own personality (especially temperament) and correspondingly on his own mood patterns and empathic understanding: blunted affect, ambivalent, parathymic (inappropriate affect), affective lability, affective incontinence, affective rigidity.

Items of Somatic States Are Easier To Define

Compared with the psychopathological item sheet, the items of the somatic state do not involve equally severe problems of definition. The rating of the item group 'disorders of appetite and libido' has to rely mostly on an intraindividual comparison.

Scaling of Items – Choosing what Criteria?

Thus, it should be clear that the operationability of many AMDP items are at least questionable. In the AMDP the process of decision for rating goes on in four steps (fig. 1) in a *'decision tree'* [2]:

1) Whether the rater is able to examine and to judge an item. Is a decision possible or not? This depends on the patient's ability or readyness to cooperate in the diagnostic interview. E.g. if a patient with catatonic schizophrenia remains mute, only the psychomotor rubric of AMDP sheet 3 can be rated. – Similar problems arise when a patient refuses answers for whatever reasons or in oligophrenia, clouded consciousness, aphasia.
2) Certainty with which a statement 'is present' or 'is not present' can be given: 'certainly present', 'presence questionable'. For similar reasons as mentioned under point 1 the certainty of the decision process whether an item is present or not may be difficult.
3) Statement concerning the presence of an item: present/not present. Such a statement has its prerequisite in clearly positive examinability (1), judgability (1), certainty of decision (2).
4) Quantification: How marked is a symptom? The problem of weighting (scaling) the items in a three-degree scale (mild, moderate and severe) is unsolved. Scaling includes at least two aspects: intensity of a symptom (which is hardly to define clearly), frequency and/or duration of a symptom. It was decided that 'intensity' should be the main criteria for scaling.

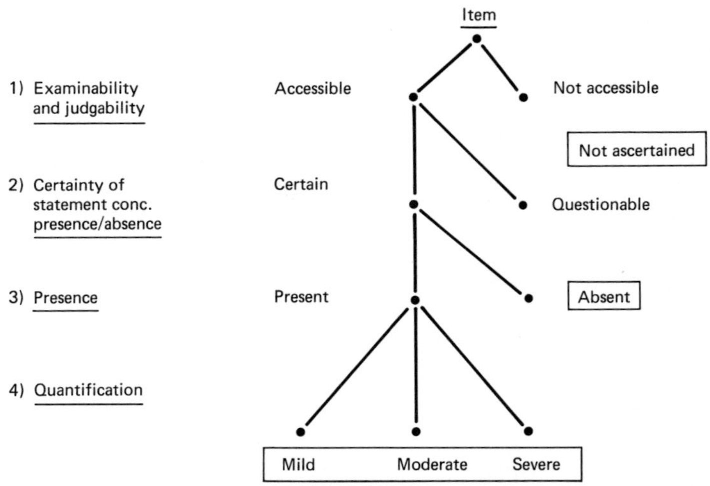

Fig. 1. AMP/ADMP decision tree.

Interview and Rating Training Makes AMDP a Useful Instrument

In spite of all the mentioned problems of the AMDP for evaluating and documenting a psychopathological state, it has proved to be a useful instrument in many institutes when applied to various categories of psychiatric patients. By special interview and rating training an acceptable degree of rater consensus can be achieved.

We established a continuous training for the residents of our institute. Once a week (for about 2 h) in a group of about 6–8 participants one of the residents interviews a patient. Afterwards an AMDP sheet on 'psychopathology' is filled out by each participant. The results are then compared, consensus and dissensus discussed. After that the style and technique of the interview is dealt with. This interrater training can easily be combined with the use of other instruments for psychopathology (e.g. depression scale). We have a further 2-hours training, stressing more the type, style, technique of first diagnostic evaluation, differential diagnostic process, psychodynamics of interview, and training in summarizing and conclusion-drawing of psychopathological state and case history. Both training types are complementary to each other. We prefer the direct life situation of interview in a small group, headed by an experienced psychiatrist. Up to now we do not use video tapes and/or the separated and to some degree always artificial situation of one-way mirror interview rooms. It would raise a lot of ethical and juridical problems complicating the patient-interviewer interaction. It proved to be helpful that staff members join the interview group: they can contribute their own observations while taking care of the patient in his hospital life, and they prevent the patient from being exposed to a completely strange group of doctors (which might be relevant for the information to be gained from him).

The AMDP may be used for the routine documentation and for research purposes. It is helpful also for training in diagnostic interviewing. Thus, it can contribute in many ways to a thorough psychopathological evaluation of patients and research sampling. That is the basis for diagnostic decisions as the prerequisite of therapeutic planning and prognostic perspectives. Careful descriptive psychopathology should also forego psychodynamic interpretation (interpretative, understanding psychopathology) as a complementary approach to deal with mental patients.

References

1a AMP-System: Manual zur Dokumentation psychiatrischer Befunde (Springer, Berlin 1971).

1b Das AMDP-System: Manual zur Dokumentation psychiatrische Befunde; 3. Aufl. (Springer, Berlin 1978).

2 Bente, D.; Engelmeier, M. P.; Heinrich, K.; Hippius, H.; Schmitt, W.: Zur Dokumentation medikamentöser Wirkungen bei der psychiatrischen Pharmakotherapie. Arzneimittel Forsch. *11:* 886–890 (1961).

3 Bleuler, E.: Dementia Praecox oder die Gruppe der Schizophrenien; in Aschaffenburg, Handbuch der Psychiatrie, spez. Teil 4, 1. Hälfte (Deuticke, Leipzig 1911).

4 Conrad, K.: Die beginnende Schizophrenie. Versuch einer Gestaltanalyse des Wahns (Thieme, Stuttgart 1958).

5 Gruhle, H. W.: Allgemeine Symptomatologie der Schizophrenie; in Bumke Handbuch der Geisteskrankheiten, vol. 9, spez. Teil V (Springer, Berlin 1932).

6 Hecker, E.: Die Hebephrenie. Virchows Arch. path. Anat. *52:* 394–429 (1871).

7 Jaspers, K.:Allgemeine Psychopathologie; VII. Aufl. (Springer, Berlin 1959).

8a Kahlbaum, K. L.: Die Gruppierung der psychiatrischen Krankheiten (Kafemann, Danzig 1863).

8b Kahlbaum, K. L.: Die Katatonie oder das Spannungsirresein (Hirschwald, Berlin 1874).

9 Kraepelin, E.: Psychiatrie. Ein Lehrbuch für Studierende und Ärzte; 8. Aufl. (Barth, Leipzig 1905–1915).

10 Lorr, M.; Klett, C.J.; McNair, D.M.; Lasuy, J.J.: Inpatient multidimensional psychiatric scale manual (Consult. Psychol. Press, Palo Alto 1963).
11 Schneider, K.: Klinische Psychopathologie (Thieme, Stuttgart 1967).
12 Wing, J.K.; Cooper, J.E.; Sartorius, N.: Measurement and classification of psychiatric symptoms. An instruction manual for the PSE and CATEGO program (Cambridge University Press, London 1974).
13 Wundt, W.: Grundriss der Psychologie (Kröner, Leipzig 1922).

C. Scharfetter, MD, Psychiatric University Hospital, Research Department, CH-8029 Zürich (Switzerland)

Mod. Probl. Pharmacopsychiat., vol. 20, pp. 55–67 (Karger, Basel 1983)

AMDP Information-Processing Systems

H. H. Stassen[a], *D. Bente*[b], *J. Feder*[b], *K. Freudenthal*[b], *A. Strauss*[c]

[a]Psychiatric University Clinic, Research Department, Zürich, Switzerland;
[b]Psychiatric University Clinic and Department of Psychophysiology, Berlin;
[c]Psychiatric University Clinic, Munich, FRG

Introduction

During the past 10 years information processing in medical research has been improved substantially due to rapidly increasing computer capacities and a permanent innovation of peripheral devices. Nevertheless, the realization of complex investigations with large amounts of data always raises new problems concerning both hardware and software aspects of information processing: data acquisition; representation of data and intrinsic structures; storage and retrieval, and interfaces to application programs.

All of these aspects depend on each other; consequently, the key goal of modern data-processing technique is an integrated system architecture which includes a special data base environment in most cases.

Obviously such an integrated system provides a greater degree of flexibility than previously available: data can be added, replaced, modified, deleted or selected by attributes for a broad range of applications. Beyond that, complex relationships may be established through the linking of cases, of facts or of properties to each other. Of course the notion of a data base as a central resource demands that much more emphasis must be placed on the internal representation of informations and their characteristics than has been in the past.

The attempt of the Association for Methodology and Documentation in Psychiatry (AMDP) group to introduce a flexible approach to information processing in psychiatry led to a standardization of collecting psychiatric data, to its representation in terms of medical informatics and to its common use in scientific research. The corresponding EDP concept was designed to meet the above-mentioned capabilities of recent computer technology and makes use of an optical mark reader (OMR) system as the central data acquisition device.

The Optical Mark Reader System

The data acquisition concept of AMDP is based on different types of documents which can be processed by an OMR. In the following a table-driven technique is presented for a computerized interpretation of the bar-marked forms, being applied in the Psychiatric University Clinic of Zürich [9]. A maximum of flexibility concerning layout and content of documents was achieved in this system by using easily edited descriptor tables. Such a descriptor table is accessible to any application program and contains all necessary details about an OMR document, including plausibility controls. It accepts up to 32 different types of data groups whereas the total number of data groups within a document is unlimited. The development of this table-driven technique could profit from experiences obtained by a first version of an OMR system installed in 1973 by the Psychiatric University Clinic of Zürich [8].

The concept provides an offline processing of documents: when a bar-marked form is read by the OMR it stores a character string on a magnetic tape appropriate to the cells marked. The conversion routine, which builds up an internal representation of the data, first transforms the character string into a 2-dimensional binary matrix representing the presence of marks on the form. In a second stage the descriptor table needed to decipher the actual document is loaded by recognizing a bar-marked identifier, preprinted in a standard position. According to the located interpretation scheme bits are combined to final values (numeric, multiple choice, etc.) forming a data record. In a third stage plausibility tests are performed which result in a detailed list of errors, remarks and missing data for subsequent reference. The complete contents of a document can either be printed in a text version or be stored into the data bank (DB) by means of the actual identification. This approach is in use since 1979 and has obvious advantages, enabling rapid implementation of new facilities and of new documents into existing applications.

The Data Base Approach

Information systems for patient care are now well-established in most hospitals and usually dispose of comfortable data management capabilities [4, 5]. But only very few systems were designed to meet the demands of medical research studies in a broad range of disciplines, because medical information systems have particularly been understood as a resource for practicing physicians or administrative users.

An information system is based on a DB, the central equipment for the representation of data and structures: i.e. facts about objects, attributes and their distinct values, relationships, associations or abstract concepts. The data integrity of such a DB is guaranteed by a data base management system (DBMS) which also performs the data retrieval, whereas a particular entity set may be referred either by an identifier or by the values of any combinaton of attributes. A DB together with an appropriate DBMS are called a data base.

The major tool for data base planning is the construction of models which represent data and structures in a manner which allows the design of application-oriented and effective systems. In practice a data model is constructed from data elements representing values of attributes of entities, and from their relationships. A data model describes only one single view of a data base and reproduces only a small subset of reality, appropriate to one application of the data base contents. The conceptual description of the data and its structure, while limited to one view, has to be powerful enough to provide a framework for the processing of the data. In order to build an integrated data base it is usually necessary to integrate a number of data models into a data base model [10]. The most often discussed data models in the literature are the relational data model, the hierarchical data model and the network model, which are the customary fundamentals of commercial systems. Besides those data base systems which guarantee a broad range of applications according to their theoretical concepts, a lot of 'local' developments have been realized. These solutions often waive a special data model but usually dispose of powerful, problem-oriented facilities of data retrieval and selection. Naturally the corresponding software is not portable in most cases.

The evolution of modern computer technology coupled with a very general availability of statistical packages led almost automatically to new applications and a successively increasing amount of data also in the field of psychiatric research. The attractiveness of data base systems for those scientific investigations increased simultaneously, due to obvious advantages in connection with the processing of research data: (1) simplified handling of large studies, even if the extend of collected informations is varying per measurement; (2) combined evaluation of data from different studies, even if overlapping, and (3) representation of relations and structures.

Moreover, no special effort is required to preserve data integrity. On the other hand, there exist several disadvantages too, which counteract to a general application of data base systems by the research community: (1) Scientific investigations are usually study-oriented (i.e. the elementary entity set identifiers are built up by the attributes 'study/group/subject/rating/...') whilst existing information systems for patient care are patient oriented. A subsequent implementation of a study-oriented approach into a well-practised data base application may raise problems. (2) Commercial data base systems are comparatively expensive, they are often provided only with a small set of data types and corresponding operations. (3) An interfacing to application programs may be difficult [6, 7], because the traditional data structure available in statistical packages is the rectangular scheme where each individual or case is represented by a single fixed length record of data.

The above-mentioned details prove the necessity of a careful discussion of information processing techniques in the broader context of project planning, for such planning may be very much affected by a data base environment.

The AMDP Information System of Zürich

The Data Base Concept

The integrated information system which has been developed by the research department of the Psychiatric University Clinic Zürich, comprises a table-driven subsystem for the interpretation of bar-marked AMDP documents, a data base system for the management of the data and a package of statistical standard programs interfacing the DB. This information system is implemented on the central computer of the university (IBM 3033/MVS) and can be initialized on any interactive terminal (TSO) as well as by batch jobs. At the moment the contents of about 20,000 AMDP forms, completed by additional information, are stored in the data bank.

```
&&START DBANK
  STUD=50.1:51.1:51.2:52.1:52.2:55.1:58.1,
  STUD=65.1:65.2:65.3:68.1:68.2,
  STUD=70.1:70.2:72.1:72.2:74.1:74.2:78.1:78.2,
  STUD=80.1:88.1:93.1:93.2:99.1:99.2:102.1,
  STUD=107.1:107.2:109.1:109.2:113.1:119.1:119.2,
  STUD=132.1:136.1:140.1:140.2,
  PERS=*ALL,RATI=*ALL,VERS=1
&&START RASTER=GEHOBEN/EUPHORISCH (AUSPR. 5,6,7)
  SYMP=69,GRAD=5,VERK=1,ANZA=300,PROT=6
&&END
```

Fig. 1. Selection of data from the AMDP DB by a DB call and its processing by the application program Raster. Several studies are selected and concatenated by a DB call using a label s, $50.1 \leq S \leq 140.2$. The following call of the program Raster determines the frequency distribution of a special symptom from the above defined set of data.

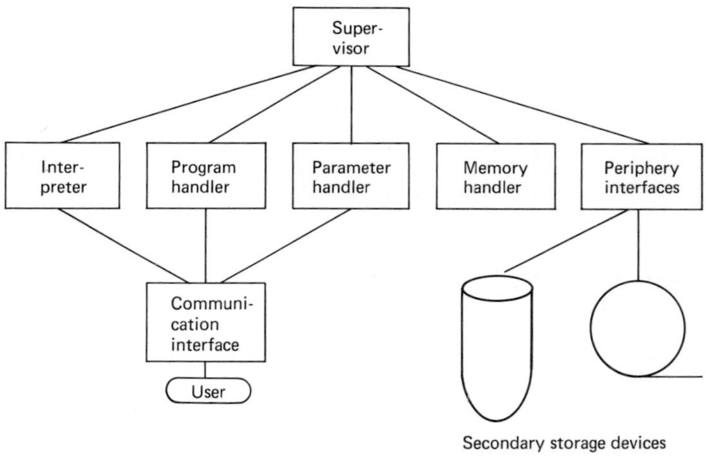

Fig. 2. Basic components of the AMDP information system.

The appropriate data base system is a special development and was designed to meet the specific demands of the local AMDP applications (e.g. psychopharmacological investigations, the course of psychiatric disorders, classification problems, computer-aided selection of diagnostic parameters, etc.). It does not satisfy all aspects of a data model of the above-mentioned types, but works exclusively with inverted lists and direct accessed files (relative block addressing). Due to this technique a good response time could be obtained for interactive operations.

All parts of the information system are controlled by a supervisor program called Master, which has its own interpreter for a format-free in-

```
UEBERSICHTSLISTE MASTER.PSYCHLIB
--------------------------------
 1  TEST        TESTLAUF FUER DIE VERWEISLISTEN
 2  LOESCHEN    LOGISCHES LOESCHEN EINES SCHLUESSELBEREICHES
 3  REORG       REORGANISATION DER VERWEISLISTEN
 4  CLEAN       PHYSIKALISCHE REORGANISATION EINES DATENFILE
 5  LADEN       LADEN VERWEISLISTEN IN WORK-BEREICH
 6  SAVE        ABSPEICHERN VERWEISLISTEN AUS WORK-BEREICH
 7  CLEAR       LOESCHEN/NORMIEREN VERWEISLISTEN
 8  DBANK       ANSCHLUSS DATENBANK
 9  GENER       UEBERNAHME DATEN VON DIGITALBAND
10  RESERVE     SPEICHERPLATZ-RESERVATION FUER AMP-BOEGEN
11  SECURE      SECURE-LAUF FUER DIE DISK-FILES
12  REWIND      ZURUECKSPULEN DATENBAND
13  KEY         DEFINITION SCHLUESSELBEGRIFF
14  BELEG       BEHANDLUNG DER AMP-BOEGEN
15  CHANGE      SPEZ-WERT-AENDERUNG IN DER AMP-DATEI
16  PHATAB      AUSWERTUNG DER SYMPTOMLISTEN
17  RANG        RANGKORRELATIONEN NACH SPEARMAN (BEI BINDUNGEN)
18  NONPAR      NICHT-PARAMETRISCHES TESTPAKET
19  PART        PARTIELLE PRODUKT-MOMENT-KORRELATIONEN
20  NORMP       NORMALITAETSPRUEFUNGEN
21  NORMA3      T-FLAECHENTRANSFORMATION, HAEUFIGKEITEN, NORMALITAET
22  PAMV        PAARWEISER MITTELWERTVERGLEICH, EINFACHE VARIANZANALYSE
23  DIFF        DIFFERENZEN VON MITTELWERTEN ABHAENGIGER STICHPROBEN
24  JONCK       VARIANZANALYSE NACH JONCKEHEERE
25  FAST        VERGLEICH VON FAKTORENSTRUKTUREN
26  HAEUGE      EINDIMENSIONALE HAEUFIGKEITSAUSZAEHLUNG
27  POWER2      ITEMANALYSE DICHOTOMER ITEMS / MULTIPLE CHOICE FORM
28  LIKERT      ITEMANALYSE FUER 3-9 ABSTUFUNGEN
29  SKAL        AUSWERTUNG VON LIKERT-SKALEN
30  ALNEV       AUSWERTUNG VON TESTS MIT 2-STUFIGER BEANTWORTUNG
31  EIGEN       EIGENWERTE EINER SYMMETRISCHEN MATRIX
32  HKOMP       HAUPTKOMPONENTENANALYSE
33  DISCR       MULTIPLE DISKRIMINANZANALYSE
34  MIS         PRODUKT-MOMENT-KORRELATIONEN
35  AVANEW      MEHRFAKTORIELLE VARIANZ-/KOVARIANZANALYSE
36  RASTER      RASTER-SUCHLAUF IN AMP-DATEI
37  LIST        LIST AMP-DATEI
```

Fig. 3. List of the subsystem Master-Psychlib which consists of DB service routines as well as of application programs.

put of parameters and data values (fig. 1). Besides the supervisor program the system consists of 5 additional components which are linked to each other by special software interfaces. All application programs communicate with the system via the same interfaces and share the installed resources (fig. 2).

Application Programs

The AMDP information system of Zürich includes a package of statistical standard programs interfacing the DB. All programs can easily be modified or extended to meet new applications. Due to this concept most investigations concerning the AMDP DB may be performed interactively without the use of any other resource (fig. 3).

```
SPEZIFIKATIONSLISTE:   PAMV
------------------------------
I4    VARI           UNDEFINIERT
I4    GRUP           UNDEFINIERT<
I4    TEST                     0   *DEFAULT-WERT
R4    ALPH                0.0500   *DEFAULT-WERT
I4    UNIT                     5   *DEFAULT-WERT
I4    DART                     1   *DEFAULT-WERT
I4    MISS                     0   *DEFAULT-WERT
A8    KENN           UNDEFINIERT<
I4    DATE                     1   *DEFAULT-WERT
I4    NSUB                     1   *DEFAULT-WERT
```

Fig. 4. List of program specifications including the actually assigned values. The application program PAMV is controled by a set of parameters whose names (VARI, GRUP, ...), types (I4, R4, A8, ...) and default values are stored in a central file. Values are assigned to parameters by instructions of the form NAME = $VALUE_1$ / $VALUE_2$ / ... where NAME stands for the parameter name and VALUE denotes an appropriate parameter value.

Application programs are called by a unique identifier within the system and all corresponding parameters are accessed analogously by problem-oriented names. No special format or ordering is required for the assignment of values to parameters (cf. examples of fig. 5). New programs are linked to the system under control of an interactive installation routine which simplifies considerably the definition of additional entities.

The system supports five independent subsystems each of which may include up to 50 programs. A single program is characterized by a set of appropriate parameters, whose attributes 'name', 'type' and 'default value' are stored in the central control file. The list of program specifications including all assigned values (both assigned implicitly by default or explicitly by instruction) is fully transparent to the user at any time (fig. 4, 5).

During the past years, the points of main effort in connection with the AMDP-System have been concentrated in Zürich to studies of psychotropic drugs (neuroleptics and antidepressants) and related problems. Investigations of such a kind follow a concept proposed by *Baumann and Rothweiler* [1] which particularly makes use of an analysis of covariance, and which has been implemented into the information system as a standard feature. Furthermore, the reliability or reproducibility of scales and categories, as well as the course of these quantities have been of special interest. Another important questioning of current research deals with classification problems and it seems to be evident that the informa-

```
00080 &&START BATCH
00090 &&START DBANK
00100    STUD=140.1:140.2,PERS=*ALL,RATI=1/2/3/4/5/6/7/8,VERS=1
00110 &&START PHATAB=DIVOX/IMIPRAMIN
00120    TEST=1/2/3,SYNDR=1
00130 &&START DBANK
00140    STUDIE=140.1,PERS=*ALL,RATI=1/2/3/4/5/6/7/8,VERS=1
00150 &&START DIFF=DIVOX
00160    VARIABLE=8,PERS=10,DART=2,MODUS=1,INDEX=1.0
00170    KENN=R1/R2/R3/R4/R5/R6/R7/R8,DATEN=12
00180 &&START DIFF=DIVOX
00190    MODUS=0,INDEX=-/1/2/3/4/5/6/7/8
00200 &&START NONPAR=DIVOX
00210    VARI=8,PERS=10,DART=2,TEST=4/6,SPEZ=0,ZWWE=0,DATEN=12,DUNN=0
00220 &&START DBANK
00230    STUDIE=140.2,PERS=*ALL,RATI=1/2/3/4/5/6/7/8,VERS=1
00240 &&START DIFF=IMIPRAMIN
00250    VARIABLE=8,PERS=10,DART=2,MODUS=1,INDEX=1.0
00260    KENN=R1/R2/R3/R4/R5/R6/R7/R8,DATEN=12
00270 &&START DIFF=IMIPRAMIN
00280    MODUS=0,INDEX=-/1/2/3/4/5/6/7/8
00290 &&START NONPAR=IMIPRAMIN
00300    VARI=8,PERS=10,DART=2,TEST=4/6,SPEZ=0,ZWWE=0,DATEN=12,DUNN=0
00310 &&START DBANK
00320    STUDIE=140.1:140.2,PERS=*ALL,RATI=1/2/3/4/5/6/7/8,VERS=1
00330 &&START NONPAR=DIVOX/IMIPRAMIN
00340    VARI=8,PERS=10,TEST=3,SPEZ=10/10,DART=2,DATEN=8,ZWWE=0,DUNN=0
00350 &&START NONPAR=DIVOX/IMIPRAMIN (DIFFERENZ ZU 1.RATING)
00360    DART=3,DATEN=7
00370 &&START DBANK
00380    STUDIE=140.1:140.2,PERS=*ALL,RATI=1,VERS=1
00390 &&START PAMV=RATING 1
00400    VARI=8,GRUP=10/10,DART=2,TEST=0,KENN=DIVOX/IMIPR
00410 &&START DBANK
00420    STUDIE=140.1:140.2,PERS=*ALL,RATI=2,VERS=1
00430 &&START PAMV=RATING 2
00440    VARI=8,GRUP=10/10,DART=2,TEST=0,KENN=DIVOX/IMIPR
00450 &&START DBANK
00460    STUDIE=140.1:140.2,PERS=*ALL,RATI=3,VERS=1
00470 &&START PAMV=RATING 3
00480    VARI=8,GRUP=10/10,DART=2,TEST=0,KENN=DIVOX/IMIPR
```

Fig. 5. Sequence of application programs (PHATAB, DIFF, NONPAR, PAMV) which are part of the standard analysis for psychotropic drugs [8]. In a first step AMDP syndromes are estimated by program PHATAB for 2 subgroups of study '140' comprising 8 ratings each (lines 90–120). In a second step both subgroups are analyzed separately (lines 130–210, 220–300) by the programs DIFF and NONPAR. In a third step a statistical comparison is performed between both subgroups (lines 310–480).

tions assessed by the AMDP instruments may contribute to the discovery of stable disease entities based on natural similarities between sets of characteristics. Such a similarity concept includes both a local similarity to distinguish fine graduations of mutual differences and a global similarity which describes structures of higher order. However, symptoms alone do not lead to a good definition of disease entities but it is necessary to consider etiologic, pathogenetic and social aspects of the individual patient too. Even though those variables are not yet sufficiently included in the assessment instruments of AMDP, no formal difficulty arises in completing the existing data by the required informations. This remarkable advantage of information systems contrasts with former data handling techniques and suggests a decision-oriented approach to the representation of data and to the operators working on it.

The above considerations show the emphasis of recent methodical investigations concerning the realm of classification problems in connection with AMDP data. The derived results may contribute to new concepts of disease entities in psychiatry, possibly defining the term 'diagnosis' which often covers a large and vague field without much precision.

Remarks

The present version of the AMDP-System is certainly not yet the optimal solution for the various aspects of information processing in psychiatry. In fully computerized applications which are based on the OMR documents of AMDP, problems may arise being due mostly to insufficient header informations. That fact led recently to some modifications within the standard headers, but at the moment these additional identifier fields are only available in the Zürich version of the AMDP-System.

Besides those technical restrictions there exist some other difficulties concerning the consistency and the comparison of logical data groups and their distinct values. These intrinsic incompatibilities have necessarily consequences for the application of similarity concepts and for investigations which aim at the discovering of entities and structures. From these details it becomes obvious that the present form of the AMDP-System is probably not a definite version but one can expect a successive improvement of this instrument.

The Data-Processing Concept of Munich

At the Psychiatric University Clinic, Munich, an information system has been established which includes all features for the acquisition, the management and the processing of clinical data. The data acquisition method is mainly based on the AMDP-System, comprising anamnestic informations, the psychopathological state at the beginning and the end of hospitalization as well as a description of the course of drug therapy.

The information system is realized on an office computer, Siemens 6640, with a 256k central memory, 2 disk drives of 40 MB storage capacity each and a line printer. This is a rather small configuration in comparison with the large-scale computer systems usually installed at universities, but it allows an optimal adaption of hardware to the specific requirements. Moreover, the operating can be done even by less trained persons.

Besides the operating system, the software distributed by the manufacturer includes a DB system, a Cobol compiler and a mask interpreter. The data acquisition has been realized by means of the mask interpreter whereas the program package for the data analysis is written in Cobol.

The DB design is based on the relational model of data and represents a finite collection of time-varying relations defined over a finite set of domains. A relation is a subset of n-tuples and is usually described as a table with distinct rows (tuples) and homogeneous columns. The ordering of rows and columns is immaterial since they are identified by content or by name respectively and not by position. The elements of a tuple are called attributes and correspond to the items of the measuring instruments, e.g. the AMDP-System. Data retrieval and application programs are supported by a special query language which disposes of the 'projection', 'join' and 'restriction' capabilities. As a result of those operations records can be counted, displayed and printed out with additional statistical informations if required. The system also provides the storage of selected data on magnetic tape. This feature allows a data analysis by means of the well-proved biostatistical program packages which are installed at the computer center of the university.

The comprehensive information system made not only the application of computing techniques to various aspects of psychiatric problems easier but also readily acceptable. The latter essentially depended on the reliability of computer hardware as well as on the comfortable data retrieval capabilities of acceptable response time.

Berlin: Recent Developments for the Processing of AMDP Data

A Graphic Approach

Two program packages Omra and Omra-T have been developed for the purpose of processing data recorded on OMR documents. They include all facilities required for the interpretation of bar-marked forms and generate files which are subsequently used for a statistical analysis.

The design of supporting software had to fulfil the following restrictions: (1) implementation on a word-oriented multiuser system; (2) it was deemed essential to use a flexible technique because several types of OMR documents were to be interpreted; (3) AMDP forms were filled up since 1968 as a routine with regard to a detailed statistical analysis.

The program package Omra was designed for the CDC 6000 series with a Scope3 or Nosbe operating system and has been realized by means of the programming languages Fortran, Algol60 and Compass. It provides a binary data input in a fixed format of 80×12 bits per record according to the OMR system.

The Omra programs also perform the plausibility controls and create packed data records which are stored on disk. For the purpose of statistical data analysis Omra disposes of a program for the generation of frequency tables as well as of an SPSS-interface. Due to this concept one can profit by the whole spectrum of statistical program packages usually available in a scientific computer center.

In 1979 a new, completely revised package Omra-T was developed in order to realize an online processing of OMR documents. This package is implemented in a computer system HP 1000 and makes use of a X-Y-Digitizer Summagraphics. The present version 1.3 supports all forms of the AMDP-System. The data acquisition is performed online by means of the digitizer with lightpen which is linked to a display terminal with keyboard. The digitizer works in pointmode and can be controlled by a Menue panel. A new form is initialized with the definition of its origin of coordinates and subsequently interpreted according to the corresponding description file. Each bar marking is displayed on the screen and each data field is checked for missing data and plausibility, in connection with which error messages are reported on the screen with detailed informations, accompanied by a striking bell signal. The contents of the document, completed by additional quantities, are organized as a data record and stored in a direct access file.

The Processing of AMDP Data on a Small Computer System

A first approach to a computerized analysis of the anamnestic, somatic and psychopathological data measured by the AMDP-System was designed 1969 for a Siemens 4004 computer system. Its realization, a program package Ampas written in Fortran [2, 3], has been a standard instrument of different users for a rather long time. It provided an offline interpretation of OMR forms which necessarily led to unpleasant turn-around times, mainly due to incorrectly processed documents. A decentralized data-processing technique, independent of the large computer centers, was found to be an optimum solution which moreover implied a reduced data protection problem. A pilot study proved that all features of the Ampas package could be adapted to a minicomputer Triumph-Adler 1100C with 32k central memory, a display terminal and a dual floppy disk drive. The data acquisition is performed interactively allowing a comfortable error correction method. Besides those capabilities, the system disposes of procedures for a selection of data by logical descriptors and of programs for a basic data analysis. An implementation of the revised version of AMDP forms from 1979 has not yet been realized, but preliminary tests showed that the relevant programs can easily be modified.

The Data-Processing Concept of Madrid, Brussels and Liège

An information system for the acquisition of all AMDP data was created at the psychiatric university clinics of Madrid, followed by Brussels and Liège. It provides an output in terms of medical forms. The processing system used in Madrid and Brussels consists of a microcomputer Commodore CBM 32K, which has several advantages: a simplified handling of hardware and no problem of response time (contrary to time sharing).

But problems arise with microcomputers as one wants multivariate statistical analyses, such as a factor analysis. Therefore, the department of psychiatry of the University of Liège combines the advantages of a microcomputer for the acquisition and edition of the data off-line (Tandy TRS-II, 64K) and the advantages of a bigger computer (IBM 4341U) through a connection to the central computer center of the University.

Conclusion

Decentralized installations of small computer systems are certainly an interesting approach to routine applications in psychiatry. Furthermore, they even allow a basic data analysis in connection with psychiatric investigations. In future this development will become much more attractive due to considerably reduced hardware costs and the benefits of recent computer technology which supports sophisticated data networks between nearly all types of computer systems.

References

1 Baumann, U.; Rothweiler, R.: Statistische Analyse von Psychopharmaka-Studien; unveröff. Merkblatt, Zürich (1973).

2 Bente, D.; Feder, J.; Siegordner, K.: Ein Programmsystem zur überregionalen Archivierung und statistischen Auswertung von AMP-Daten. Arzneimittel-Forsch. *20:* 913–915 (1970).

3 Bente, D.; Feder, J.: Ampas-Archivierung und Auswertung psychiatrischer Daten. Data Praxis D 14/4113 (Siemens Bereich Datenverarbeitung, München 1971).

4 Blomer, S.: Vergleich von Datenbankkonzepten und ihre Realisierung in praktisch verwendeten Datenbanksystemen im Hinblick auf medizinische Anwendungen. Statistical Software Newsletter *89* (1980).

5 Egmond, J. van; Vries Robbe, P. F. de; Levy, A. H.: Information systems for patient care (North-Holland, Amsterdam 1976).

6 Greis, J.: Eine Schnittstelle zwischen dem Datenbanksystem RAMIS und dem Statistiksystem SAS, Statistical Software Newsletter *1* (1980).

7 Kuhnert, A.; Blomer, R. J.; Haux, R.; Zeh, T.: Möglichkeiten der Realisierung einer Schnittstelle bei Datenbanksystemen und statistischen Auswertungssystemen. Statistical Software Newsletter *1* (1980).

8 Scheidegger, P.: AMP-Wandelprogramme; unveröffentlichtes Benützerhandbuch, Zürich (1977).

9 Stassen, H. H.; Guenter, R.: Das Programmsystem MASTER. PSYCHLIB Version 6.1; unveröffentlichtes Benützerhandbuch, Zürich (1982).

10 Wiederhold, G.: Database design (McGraw-Hill, New York 1977).

H. H. Stassen, Psychiatrische Universitätsklinik, Forschungsdirektion, Postfach 68, CH-8029 Zürich 8(Switzerland)

Factor Structure

Mod. Probl. Pharmacopsychiat., vol. 20, pp. 68–73 (Karger, Basel 1983)

Diagnostic Classification Based on the AMDP-System

P. Berner

Department of Psychiatry, University of Vienna, Vienna, Austria

Hempel's [1961] statement on the fact that 'psychiatry lacks one of the requirements of a science: a framework of concepts with agreed referents, understood in the same sense by all', is still valid today. This is illustrated by the fact that international psychiatry is today confronted with two important, competing, classification systems, i.e. ICD-9 and DSM III, and that an entire range of different diagnostic criteria which, in spite of some overlapping, diverge considerably, are used for research purposes. In this situation, the contribution toward improvement of diagnostic assignment offered by the Association for Methodology and Documentation in Psychiatry (AMDP) system can be assessed by calling to mind the fact that in all branches of medicine, the establishment of a clinical diagnosis generally proceeds in the following manner [*Debray,* 1969].

A first step consists, in principle, in an unbiased collection of abnormal phenomena which the patient exhibits at present, or has previously shown.

The second step represents a screening of the symptoms identified in step one in order to select those that independently or in a characteristic combination point to one or – with greater frequency – to several nosological entities. In the latter case, a third step must be added in which the differential diagnosis is established by utilizing not symptomatological but additional information such as laboratory findings, anamnestic data on exposure to toxic substances, etc. The problems involved in the first step do not differ essentially, in psychiatry, from those encountered in other fields of medicine. In the second step toward diagnosis, however, psychiatry faces obstacles not so frequently met with in most of the other medical disciplines, in which the choice of those symptoms to which a diagnostic significance can be attributed is reached on the basis of a 'savoir medical' [*Debray,* 1969], a knowledge acquired by medical science on the basis of manifest relations between certain symptoms or syndromes and specific etiologies or pathogeneses. In the case of many mental abnormalities, the significance attributed to symptoms or syndromes cannot be controlled by etiological or pathogenetic references. The symptom reduction effectuated in this step is oriented on hypothetical nosological entities which vary considerably from school to school. The problems encountered at the second diagnostical step also reduce the efficacy of the third one: if a psychopathological syndrome is identified by means of a hypothetical nosological entity without the possibility of positive etiological proof, only the evidence of an etiology other than the supposed one retains a differential diagnostic value. Since etiology can convincingly be asserted almost exclusively by somatic findings, differential diagnosis is reduced to the statement that the syndrome stands for the assigned diagnosis unless a plausible causal relation to an organic disturbance is revealed.

Supportive arguments for the nosological assignment of the 'functional disorders', for which possibilities of objective verification are still lacking, may in this situation be arrived at only by tracing indirect indications. One of these indications finds its basis in the assumption that the 'diseases' distinguished by the nosological system referred to differ by evolutional and diagnostic criteria: as long as a cross-section diagnosis by means of objective biological tests is not possible, the observation of the course of the disorder may attribute to one specific diagnostic assignment a higher probability than to others. In an attempt to arrive at a diagnosis without protracted observation of the illness course, one may search for criteria as for instance genetic findings, constantly evident correlation between certain psychological traumatizing factors and distinct psychopathology, or favorable response to specific therapies, regularly observed in one type of mental disorder and not in others. These are four possibilities to identify, in a cross-section examination, signs pointing to one of the hypothetical nosological entities contained in the system used: (1) The identification of symptoms or syndromes constantly correlated with the course considered significant for the 'disease' in question. (2) The proof that persons exhibiting a specific symptomatology have among their blood-relations patients presenting symptoms of the same nature. (3) Identification of precise symptoms or syndromes, making their appearance exclusively in connection with specific psychologically traumatizing events or situations. (4) The evidence that a precise symptomatological class responds regularly in the same way to certain therapies.

These possibilities of indirect verification of the hypothetical nosological concept in use are actually widely applied. Up to the present, however, no classification fully satisfies either one or several of the four requirements. Attempts to improve the conventional diagnostic assignments or to exchange them in favor of a new classification are thus a main topic of research in psychiatry. The role of the AMDP-System in this ongoing process will be exposed in reference to each of the three diagnostic steps already delineated.

As mentioned before, the first step of the diagnostic process focuses on an unbiased collection of symptoms. During the last decades, psychiatry has made considerable progress in this direction by developing data recording systems which avoid the neglection of certain pathological phenomena, a common fault in purely narrative case histories. A further basis for adequate utilization of the observations made during step one is a precise definition of the items contained in the assessment documents, which must be understood in the same sense by all raters. As more extensively described in other chapters of this book, the AMDP-System has proved an excellent instrument to meet these requirements. Its assessment documents oblige the examining psychiatrist to pay attention to the entire psychopathology a patient might exhibit and to control his own observations as to comprehensiveness and degree of certainty, by the decisions required of him through the necessity of rating each item.

As an instrument conceived for broad clinical use, it is comprehensive enough to circumvent the pitfalls of shorter rating scales which, although also attempting to avoid the bias inherent in purely descriptive registration of observations, enhance on the other hand another selective procedure which may impair the further stages of diagnostic process by reducing the 'matrix' from which the nosological assignment must be extracted. The glossary provided by the AMDP-System offers refined definitions of psychopathological terms, leading to a high degree of interrater reliability which may be further improved through rating exercises carried through with the personnel operating the system.

The second step in the diagnostic process serves in principle two purposes. The first one aims to define correlations between certain symptoms and thus to identify syndromic constellations. In serving this purpose, factor analyses of the psychopathological and somatic symptoms rated by the AMDP-System have contributed considerably to classification in psychiatry by identifying distinct syndromes. *Baumann* [1974] thus derived a set of factors ranging from 2 to 9. The 2-factor solution permits the distinction between a depressive and a paranoid-hallucinatory syndrome. A hostility factor has furthermore been extracted in the intermediate solutions, representing a third syndrome of clinical importance. An intercorrelation of the nine syndromes led to the identification of the following nine clinically meaningful factors: apathy, hallucinatory syndrome, hostility, manic syndrome, somatic depressive syndrome, paranoid syndrome, catatonic syndrome, retarded depressive syndrome and hypochondriasis. Other important examples for the identification of syndromes by use of the AMDP-System have been provided by *Mombour* et al. [1973], *Angst* et al. [1979], *Bobon* et al. [1982] and others [for more citations, see *Baumann* et al. and *Pietzcker* et al., this volume].

These examples demonstrate that through the use of statistical methods, the AMDP-System provides a basis for identification of syndromes which may prove more objective than those obtained by a synopsis of observations not controlled by the use of standardized data records.

The second purpose pursued in step two of the diagnostic process is to single out symptoms or syndromes pointing to distinct nosological entities. In the case of functional disorders for which, as already mentioned, possibilities of objective verification for the assignment are still lacking, assignment criteria can only be listed more or less arbitrarily. During the last decade there has been a strong tendency to abandon the synoptic diagnoses obtained by clinical intuition and to render the process of assignment more explicit by the use of appropriate algorithms generally called 'diagnostic criteria'. Three different ways to conceptualize such algorithms may be distinguished.

The first one consists in a purely pragmatical approach as introduced for example by *Schneider* [1980] when he formulated his 'first-rank' and 'second-rank' symptoms for the diagnosis of schizophrenia.

The second may be called 'theory-oriented' and had its first representative in *Bleuler* [1979] whose diagnostic procedure relies on a theoretical concept of the illness process which led him to the establishment of a symptom hierarchy, distinguishing between 'basic' and 'accessory' symptoms in schizophrenic disorders. One more example of a theory-oriented establishment of diagnostic algorithms is the hierarchial semiology or *Schichtregel* [*Jaspers*, 1959] stipulating that schizophrenic features deprive manic-depressive symptoms of their diagnostic significance. The third approach is purely empirical and has, in the field of functional psychoses, its original sources in the observations on schizo-affective psychoses by *Kasanin* and his successors and in the publications on schizophreniform psychoses emanating from the Scandinavian school. These empirical algorithms generally encompass a variety of symptomatological and non-symptomatological indicators considered to be significant for the assignment to a specific diagnosis. Concerning the subdivision of functional psychoses, for example, indicators for a poor prognosis determine the attribution to schizophrenia whereas data empirically correlated with a good prognosis result in the diagnosis of an affective disorder. Empirically constituted diagnostic criteria frequently involve psychopathological elements of pragmatical or theory-oriented algorithms in various combinations, and eventually reverse *Jaspers'* [1959] semiological hierarchy. Some of them include time criteria.

Some authors have developed 'short forms' of the AMDP-System, for instance for schizophrenic or depressive symptomatology, based on factor analysis [*Woggon and Dittrich,* 1979]. Since the background of the AMDP-System has its main sources in *Bleuler's* and *Schneider's* psychopathology, these subscales are algorithms representing a combination of pragmatical and theory-oriented approaches.

At present, the AMDP-System does not yet contain all necessary elements for application of the many diagnostic criteria representing the empirical approach currently in use, mainly in the USA. The reason for this is of a historical nature: the AMDP-System was originally conceptualized as an instrument for therapy evaluation and was used prior to the establishment of the Anglo-Saxon diagnostic criteria. However, since the AMDP-System covers most of the areas from which those criteria are derived – i.e. demographic data, life events, psychopathological symptoms and somatic signs – it should not be difficult to complete the system, which could then serve as a matrix for application of the prevailing algorithms used by other researchers. The embodiment of supplementary items into the assessment documents seems to be of primary importance. The operators of the AMDP-System would thus be enabled to compare different methods of classification in the sense of a 'poly-diagnostic' approach [*Helmchen,* 1980; *Berner and Katschnig,* in press]. This could be an important contribution to the task of investigation as to which classification method proves to be of the highest validity within the verification procedure taking place in step three of the diagnostic process.

In the case of functional disorders, the third diagnostic step, as already mentioned, pertains to the correlation between a nosological class established in step two, a specific illness course, genetic findings, psychological traumata, or treatment response. The AMDP-System is well equipped to evaluate the course of a disturbance and its response to defined treatments by means of repeated ratings. It includes also rating possibilities for genetic data and stressful life events, the latter ones however still requiring further elaboration.

Furthermore, the different areas of information included in the AMDP assessment documents cover most of the 'axes' or 'dimensions' of the multiaxial or multidimensional classifications currently in use. In similarity to the earlier comments on diagnostic algorithms, the inclusion of some additional elements into the present version of the AMDP-System could elevate it to represent a 'polyvalent' diagnostic instrument, benefiting the first step of the dignostic process and utilizable by different schools.

References

Angst, A.; Dittrich, A.; Woggon, B.: Reproduzierbarkeit der Faktorenstruktur des AMP-Systems. Int. Pharmacopsychiat. *14:* 319–324 (1979).

Baumann, U.: Diagnostische Differenzierungsfähigkeit von Psychopathologieskalen. Arch. Psychiat. NervKrankh. *219:* 89–103 (1974).

Berner, P.; Katschnig, H : Principles of 'multiaxial' classification in psychiatry as a basis of modern methodology; in Helgason, Methodology in evaluation of psychiatric treatment (in print).

Bleuler, E.: in Lehrbuch der Psychiatrie; 14. Aufl. (Springer, Berlin 1979).

Bobon, D.; Mormont, C ; Doumont, A.; Mirel, J.; Bonhomme, P.; Ansseau, M.; Pellet, J.; Pull, C.; De Buck, R.; Gernay, P.; Mormont, I.; Lang, F.; Lejeune, J.; Bronckart, C.; Frenckell, R. von: Analyse factorielle de la révision française de l'échelle AMDP. Résultats d'une étude internationale de 388 cas. Acta psychiat. belg. *82:* 371–389 (1982).

Debray, H. R.: Echelles d'appréciation: contrôle et comparaison des diagnostics psychiatriques à l'aide d'ordinateurs. Confront. psychiat. *4:* 73–86 (1969).

Helmchen, H.: Multiaxial systems of classification. Types of axes. Acta psychiat. scand. *61:* 43–55 (1980).

Hempel, C. G.: Introduction to problems of taxonomny; in Zubin, Field studies in the mental disorders, pp. 3–22 (Grune & Stratton, New York 3–22, 1961).

Jaspers, K.: Allgemeine Psychopathologie; 7. Aufl. (Springer, Berlin 1959).

Mombour, W.; Gammel, G.; Zerssen, D. von; Heyse, H.: Die Objektivierung psychiatrischer Syndrome durch multifaktorielle Analyse des psychopathologischen Befundes. Nervenarzt *44:* 352–358 (1973).

Schneider, K.: Klinische Psychopathologie; 12. Aufl. (Thieme, Stuttgart 1980).

Woggon, B.; Dittrich, A.: Konstruktion übergeordneter AMP-Skalen: 'manisch-depressives' und 'schizophrenes' Syndrom. Int. Pharmacopsychiat. *14:* 325–337 (1979).

Prof. Dr. P. Berner, Department of Psychiatry, University of Vienna,
Lazarettgasse 14, A-1097 Vienna (Austria)

Mod. Probl. Pharmacopsychiat., vol. 20, pp. 74–87 (Karger, Basel 1983)

Syndromes and Scales in the AMP-System[1]

U. Baumann[a], *A. Pietzcker*[b], *B. Woggon*[c]

[a]Department of Psychology, University of Salzburg, Austria
[b]Department of Psychiatry, Free University of Berlin, Berlin, FRG
[c]Department of Psychiatry, Research Division, University of Zürich, Zürich, Switzerland

General Introduction

According to *von Zerssen* [23, p. 508], a syndromatology of psychic disorders must proceed from 'the joint occurrence of symptoms without consideration of their origins as the highest principle of organization'. Along with the more clinically oriented procedures, increasingly more mathematical-statistical procedures for the construction of syndromes have been used in the last 20 years, especially factor analysis. Empirical studies in which syndromes are worked out by means of mathematical-statistical methods have two purposes: (1) The *examination of syndromes* which are postulated as a result of clinical experience. In this case one is as a rule content with a discussion of the factors without specifying rules by which one would calculate the corresponding syndrome scores in the individual case. (2) Authors strive for a more far-reaching purpose that not only examines clinical syndromes, but also makes suggestions as to *syndrome scales*. Thus, the scales based on factor analysis are further evaluated by means of the methods of classical test theory (item-test correlation, distribution form, intercorrelation of the scales, reliability coefficients). Scales thus formed are suitable for use in widely varied research areas (e.g. psychopharmaca studies), since the parameters of the scales are satisfactorily characterized.

The research concerning the Association for Methodology and Documentation in Psychiatry (AMP) system (1st and 2nd editions) has been

[1] Dipl.-Psych. *R. D. Stieglitz* was a great help during the preparatory work for this article, for which he is especially thanked.

concentrated on studies which reexamine syndromes. There are three suggestions as to scale construction (*AMDP* [24]):

AMP-System [1]. Syndromes by means of factor analysis. First-order factors[2]: *Mombour* et al. [13], *Baumann* [3, 4], *Wegscheider* [17], *Sulz-Blume* et al. [15], *Gebhardt* et al. [8]. Second-order factors: *Baumann and Angst* [5], *Woggon and Dittrich* [20].

AMP-System [1]. Construction of scales with item analyses. First-order factors: *Baumann* [4], *Gebhardt* et al. [8]; second-order factors: *Woggon and Dittrich* [20], *AMDP* [24].

Methodological Preliminary Remarks as to the Comparability of Solutions

The use of factor analysis as a method of structuring data involves different methodological problems, which cannot be described in detail here. The comparability of solutions (syndromes) gained from different studies depends upon the similarity of the methodological procedures chosen by the individual authors. Different procedures are possible in these and other points:

Scaling of Symptoms. The classification of symptoms can be reduced to two categories: 'symptom present' ≡ 1 and 'absent' ≡ 0. In the statistical processing, however, the following pragmatic solution is mostly chosen: not present ≡ 0, mild ≡ 1, moderate ≡ 2, severe ≡ 3. The additional categories of the earlier AMP System 'doubtful' and 'not assessable' – summed up in the later AMDP-System in 'not ascertained' – can be considered as missing data or, for pragmatic reasons, be evaluated as 'not present'. The different authors chose the scale 0/1/2/3, whereas the seldom occurring markings in the category 'not ascertained' were also counted in the category 'not present'.

Choosing the Symptoms to Be Analyzed. When analyzing clinical data, one is usually confronted with the problem of having mostly rare

[2] The factor solution by *von Cranach* et al. [7] and *Tegeler* et al. [16] are not considered in the following since homogenous samples of patients were used, thus limiting the solution's validity. Also not considered is a study by *Hentschel* et al. [9] who made a joint analysis of the AMP and the Inpatient Multidimensional Psychiatric Scale (IMPS).

events. The factor analysis can then lead to syndromes which are only relevant for small partial samples [11]. For this reason, a cut-off criterion is often set (percentage of the symptoms present), which a symptom may not fall short of in order to be included in the factor analysis. Different limits are used in the individual studies. Also, the somatic symptoms are included in the analysis sometimes complete, sometimes without neurological symptoms, and sometimes without 'further somatic symptoms' and neurological symptoms.

Sample Selection. The individual analyses are based on differently constructed samples (compare original literature), especially with regard to the characteristics: sex, ICD-diagnosis and date of rating.

Choice of Marker Items. Different criteria are used in choosing the symptoms which help in interpreting a factor. Often, factor loads greater than 0.3 or 0.4 are interpreted. Sometimes it is required that a marker item loads minimally on the other factors ($d \geq$ critical value) or that it is specific for the factor ($a^2/h^2 \geq 0.50$).

In reference to the *factor extraction method* (main components analysis with 1 in the diagonal) and the method of *rotation* (orthogonal varimax rotation) the individual studies do not differ.

Overall differences can be found in various points of procedure according to author, so that the divergencies in the solutions can also be traced back to differing methodological procedures.

First-Order Syndromes (Factors)

The first-order syndromes are based on various samples (compare original literature). As to the number of interpreted factors *Baumann* [3, 4], *Gebhardt* et al. [8], *Mombour* et al. [13], *Sulz-Blume* et al. [15] each found 9 factors, whereas *Wegscheider* [17] found 12. The variance accounted for by the factors lies between 24 and 64%. Table I gives an overview of the different solutions.

The degree of similarity between various syndrome solutions is not established by the identity or similarity of the syndrome names, since different things can be labelled identically. Therefore, empirical studies are necessary in which the different syndromes are compared. As a result of methodological differences in the various studies, the factor structures cannot be compared with each other. Instead, only the estimated factor values can be compared (calculation of scores based on the marker items). *Pietzcker* et al. [14] and *Woggon* [19] carried out such correlation studies using two independent samples (*Woggon* n = 981, *Pietzcker* et al. n = 2269). In considering the results, it must be required that scales stemming from different solutions, but which define the same construct, correlate at least to the extent of a parallel test correlation (*Lienert* [10]: $r \geq 0.80$). The intercorrelation with construct-unrelated scales should be considerably less.

An empirical comparison of the five syndrome solutions (table I) shows the following results:

1. Sample-Independent Syndromes
(Present in all Five Solutions)

Apathy (e.g. retarded, lack of drive): the corresponding syndromes correlate highly with one exception ($r \geq 0.77$). *Hostility* (e.g. aggressiveness, dysphoria): all intercorrelations are above 0.85. *Manic syndrome* (e.g. increased drive, excessive social contact): all intercorrelations are above 0.84.

2. Sample-Independent Syndromes
(Present in Four Solutions)

Psycho-Organic Syndrome (e.g. Disturbances of Orientation, Disturbances of Attention and Immediate Memory). The corresponding scales correlate with $r \geq 0.78$. As a result of the composition of the sample, no corresponding syndrome was found in the sample of *Baumann* [3,4].

Autonomic Syndrome (e.g. Nausea, Dizziness). Contrary to *Baumann* [3, 4], all other authors have included the – in part seldomly occurring – somatic symptoms in their analyses. This leads to a syndrome called hypochondriasis by *Mombour* et al. [13], autonomic syndrome by *Wegscheider* [17] and *Gebhardt* et al. [8], and somatic-autonomic syndrome by *Sulz-Blume* et al. [15]. The different solutions correlate with each other at $r \geq 0.78$. The syndrome hypochondriasis of *Baumann* [3,4] has more in common with the depression syndrome than with the identically named syndrome by *Mombour* et al. [13]. The somatic syndrome by *Wegscheider*

Table I. AMP factor analyses by different authors

General notation	Author, place, sample				
	Baumann [3, 4] Zürich Psychiatric Clinic n=351	*Mombour* et al. [13] Munich MPI n=454	*Wegscheider* [17][1] Berlin Psychiatric Clinic n=1,066	*Sulz-Blume* et al. [15] Munich University n=1,199	*Gebhardt* et al. [8] Berlin Psychiatric Clinic n=2,269
Apathy syndrome (Apathisches Syndrom)	*	*	*	*	*
Manic syndrome (Manisches Syndrom)	*	*	*	*	*
Hostility syndrome (Hostilitäts-Syndrom)	*	aggressive touchiness (aggressive Gereiztheit)	*	*	*
Psycho-organic syndrome (Psychoorganisches Syndrom)		*	*	*	*
Autonomic syndrome (Vegetatives Syndrom)		hypochondriasis (hypochondrisches S.)	*	somatic-autonomic s. (somatisch-vegetatives S.)	somatic s. (vegetatives S.)
Depressive syndrome (Depressives Syndrom)	retarded-depressive s. (gehemmt-depressives S.)	*	*	*	*

	somatic-depressive s. (somatisch- depressives S.) hypochondriasis (hypochondrisches S.)				
Paranoid-hallucinatory syndrome (Paranoid-halluzinatorisches Syndrom)	hallucinatory s. (halluzinatorisch-desintegratives S.) paranoid s. (paranoides S.)	*	paranoid syndrome (paranoides S.)	*	*
Catatonic/stuporous syndrome (Katatones/Stuporöses Syndrom)	catatonic s. (katatones S.)	'in-need-of-care' s. (Pflegebedürftigkeit)	'in-need-of-care' s. (Pflegebedürftigkeit) stuporous-retarded s. (stuporös-gehemmtes S.)	catatonic s. (katatones S.)	stuporous s. (stuporöses S.)
Obsessive-compulsive syndrome (Zwangssyndrom)		phobic-anancastic s. (phobisch-anankastisches S.)	anancastic s. (anankastisches S.)	*	*

* Scale exists in the concerning solution; identical with the general notation.

[1] Two additional syndromes were only found by *Wegscheider* [17]: Somatic syndrome (Somatisches Syndrom), Rater factor (Beurteilerfaktor)

et al. [17] covaries little with the autonomic syndrome, since it includes neurological and vegetative symptoms.

3. Sample-Independent Solutions, in which a Few Individual Syndromes Are Split into Partial Syndromes

Depressive Syndromes (e.g. Hopelessness, Feelings of Inadequacy). With the exception of the Zürich sample [3, 4], in which the depressive symptomatology is represented by three syndromes (somatic-depressive syndrome, retarded depressive syndrome, hypochondriasis), one syndrome each is postulated in the remaining four samples. In these four samples, the corresponding syndromes correlate at $r \geq 0.78$. Of the Zürich solution, the retarded depressive syndrome corresponds most closely to the depressive syndromes found in the other samples ($r \geq 0.69$). However, the somatic depressive syndromes and hypochondriasis also show considerable correlations with the depressive syndromes of the other 4 samples. The splitting of the depressive symptomatology found in the Zürich sample is a result of the composition of the sample, and is probably only of interest for special studies. In all other cases, one depressive syndrome is sufficient.

Paranoid-Hallucinatory Syndrome (e.g. Delusional Perception, Thought Insertions). Here again we have, with the exception of the Zürich sample in which two syndromes are found (hallucinatory syndrome, paranoid syndrome, which, however, correlate with each other at $r = 0.52–0.75$), one syndrome each. In many cases, *one* syndrome should suffice. The corresponding syndromes correlate at $r \geq 0.84$, respectively.

4. Comparable Syndromes, which, however, Are Dependent upon the Sample

Although the following two syndromes have been found in several samples, syndromes corresponding to one another show correlations concentrating around the middle values, so that identical names do not cover identical construct areas.

Catatonic Syndrome/Stuporous Syndrome (e.g. Mutism, Lack of Self-Care). *Baumann* [3, 4] and *Sulz-Blume* et al. [15] postulate a catatonic syndrome, and *Gebhardt* et al. [8] a stuporous syndrome, while *Mombour* et al. [13] sum up similar symptoms under the syndrome: 'lack of self-care'.

Wegscheider [17], on the other hand, found two syndromes: 'lack of self-care' and stuporous syndrome. The correlations, which in part are in the middle range, indicate that the various syndromes cover similar phenomena. However, contrary to the syndromes discussed above in paragraphs 1–3, we are not dealing here with a construct identical for all syndromes.

Obsessive-Compulsive Syndrome (e.g. Obsessive Thoughts, Compulsive Impulses). With the exception of the Zürich sample, in which as a result of the rareness of these symptoms no syndrome was postulated, the remaining four studies each found an obsessive compulsive syndrome. The respective syndromes comprise, however, only three to four symptoms, which leads to low reliability of the syndrome. Therefore, it is not surprising that in part the identically named syndromes show only low correlations with each other.

The factors discussed by *Wegscheider* [17], 'judgment factor' and 'somatic factor', are not identifiable in the other solutions and appear to be sample-specific.

The sample independency of the syndromes can be examined using samples from different clinics (see above). There is also the possibility, however, of evaluating sample-independency by using partial samples of the same clinic. *Gebhardt* et al. [8] evaluated their data thus, and were able to identify the nine syndromes in all partial samples. In a more recent sample, *Angst* et al. [2] subjected *Baumann's* [3, 4] nine syndromes to a cross-validation (comparison of factor structure according to Fischer-Roppert). The hypochondriasis could not be reproduced in this study, while the paranoid syndrome stayed just under the critical similarity score of Ae = 0.8 usually required. The remaining seven scales could be reproduced.

Second-Order Syndromes (Factors)

Since first-order factors are as a rule interdependent, one strives to form factors of a higher order. Second-order factors can be obtained by way of two procedures [5]: (1) Extraction of only a few factors (e.g. two or three) using data which is otherwise used to obtain primary factors. (2)

Analysis of the intercorrelations of primary scales; i.e. factor analysis with intercorrelating primary scales.

Baumann and Angst [5], as well as *Woggon and Dittrich* [20], have carried out factor analytical studies which deal with second-order factors. *Baumann and Angst* [5] carried out the factor analysis both because of the intercorrelations of the 86 symptoms and the primary scales (first-order factors). In the first case, a two-factor solution (using Varimax rotation) was chosen for the highest organizational level with the syndromes: 'depressive syndrome' and 'paranoid-hallucinatory syndrome'. The intercorrelations of the nine primary scales also lead to a two-factor solution: manic-depressive syndrome (manic syndrome/apathy retarded-depressive syndrome, hypochondriasis) and paranoid-hallucinatory syndrome (hallucinatory syndrome, catatonic syndrome, paranoid syndrome). In their newer studies concerning the AMP-System, *Woggon and Dittrich* [20] found two overall syndromes, which they call 'manic-depressive syndrome' and 'schizophrenic syndrome'. These two syndromes proved – contrary to the first-order system – to be very stable in their factorial structure over time (similarity coefficients above 0.9) [21].

Test-Statistical Analyses of the Syndrome Scales

If the syndromes found are to be used for further investigations, test-statistical analyses are necessary: item analyses, information pertaining to reliability, validity and intercorrelation of scales. Validity studies are dealt with elsewhere, and will not be discussed at this point. The reliability of AMP Scales is also only treated briefly here (compare the chapter on the interrater study concerning AMP symptoms).

Studies of First-Order Syndrome Scales. Farther reaching information is available on the syndromes by *Baumann* [4] and *Gebhardt* et al. [8]. Table II presents a summary of the most important results.

Most of the scales by *Baumann* [3, 4] and *Gebhardt* et al. [8] show an adequate middle-range item-test correlation, wherein the consistency proves to be satisfactory. In *Baumann's* [3, 4] study, in particular hypochondriasis and the catatonic syndrome show less favorable parameters in consistency. For *Gebhardt* et al. [8] this is true especially for the scale which includes only three symptoms: 'obsessive-compulsive syndrome'.

Table II. Scale length (k), average item-test correlation coefficients ($\bar{r}_{it}$, part-whole corrected), internal consistency (Cronbach α) of the first-order scales by *Baumann* [3,4], *Gebhardt* et al. [8] and of the second-order scales by *Woggon and Dittrich* [20]

Baumann [3,4]				*Gebhardt* et al. [8]				*Woggon and Dittrich* [20]			
scale	k	$\bar{r}_{it}$	α	scale	k	$\bar{r}_{it}$	α	scale	k	$\bar{r}_{it}$	α
Apathy s.	7	0.52	0.80	paranoid-hallucinatory s.	15	0.49	0.86	manic-			
Hallucinatory s.	10	0.43	0.77	manic s.	11	0.46	0.81	depressive s.	27	0.49	0.91
Hostility	9	0.51	0.80	psycho-organic s.	9	0.50	0.80	schizo-			
Manic s.	9	0.54	0.83	depressive s.	9	0.42	0.74	phrenic s.	25	0.46	0.89
Somatic-depressive s.	8	0.42	0.73	apathetic s.	8	0.41	0.73				
Paranoid s.	10	0.50	0.81	hostile s.	6	0.43	0.69				
Catatonic s.	9	0.38	0.68	stuporous s.	6	0.41	0.66				
Retarded-depressive s.	9	0.50	0.81	somatic s.	9	0.32	0.63				
Hypochondriasis	7	0.35	0.64	compulsive s.	3	0.40	0.55				

Lower in consistency are also the stuporous syndrome, autonomic syndrome and hostility. Whereas the individual scales by *Gebhardt* et al. [8] are relatively independent of each other (no correlations above 0.35), middle-to higher-range correlations can be found in part for the nine scales by *Baumann* [4]. Intercorrelations (up to 0.75) occur especially between the paranoid syndrome and the hallucinatory syndrome, as well as between the somatic depressive syndrome, retarded depressive syndrome and hypochondriasis. These correlations question the differential significance of the scales for general studies. *Baumann* [3, 4] and *Gebhardt* et al. [8] each transformed the extremely negatively skewed score distributions using logarithmic transformation into T-scores (M = 50, s = 10) in order to establish a standard measure.

Studies Concerning Second-Order Syndrome Scales. Woggon and Dittrich [20] carried out test-statistical analyses of their suggested overall syndromes (table II). The middle-range item-test correlations, and as a result the consistencies are satisfactory. However, the two scales still correlate at r = –0.34.

Information as to the Reliability of the Scales

Along with the consistency of the scales (see above), the interrater reliability deserves special interest. Also, information as to retest-reliability is revealing, insofar as it deals with shorter time intervals. In reliability studies two aspects must be differentiated: numeric agreement (calculated with kappa) and agreement as to the rank-order of the scale scores insofar as several patients are tested (calculated with rank-order correlation) (table III).

The retest coefficients (rho and kappa respectively) of the first-order syndrome scales are high in the overall sample as well as in the partial samples [18, 22]. The short time span between the two ratings, and the fact that the same raters were involved both times, most likely help influence this (in clinical retest studies rather rare) finding.

Rater agreement (2 raters each; table II) [6] is lowest on the rank-order for the hostility, manic syndrome and somatic-depressive syndrome scales. The numeric agreement is low especially for the somatic-depressive syndrome. An interrater study by *Maurer-Groeli* [12] using a homogeneous sample with only 2 raters cannot be discussed here.

Table III: Reliability coefficients of the scales by *Baumann* [3,4]

	Number of items	Retest (24 h) *Woggon* et al. [22] heterogenous sample (n=80)		Interrater *Baumann and Woggon* [6] n=48	
		rho	kappa	rho	kappa
1 Apathy syndrome	7	0.85	0.87	0.78	0.89
2 Hallucinatory syndrome	10	0.88	0.90	0.68	0.73
3 Hostility	9	0.82	1.00	0.55	0.78
4 Manic syndrome	9	0.72	0.87	0.64	0.84
5 Somatic-depressive syndrome	8	0.83	0.84	0.64	0.56
6 Paranoid syndrome	10	0.87	0.90	0.72	0.89
7 Catatonic syndrome	9	0.90	0.93	0.77	0.67
8 Retarded-depressive syndrome	9	0.87	1.00	0.68	0.73
9 Hypochondriasis	7	0.83	0.90	0.87	0.78
Median		0.85	0.90	0.68	0.78

rho = agreement of rank-order; kappa=numerical agreement ($r_{tt} = 0.8$).

In the overall scales by *Woggon and Dittrich* [20], the retest correlations (rho and kappa), having values above 0.86, are of higher stability than the primary scales. The judgment agreement is sufficient (rho ≥ 0.76, kappa ≥ 0.75). No information is available on the scales by *Gebhardt* et al. [8].

Consequences of the AMDP Revision for Scale Formation

The revision of the AMP-System has led to the removal or modification in the AMDP-System of various symptoms which had served as marker items for individual syndromes. The syndrome scales of the revised AMDP version are described in the next chapter by *Pietzcker* et al.

Conclusion

The syndrome analyses carried out so far in the AMP-System have shown that comparable syndromes are identifiable in different samples, and that these syndromes satisfy test-statistical criteria. Therefore, it seems justifiable to carry out evaluations – not only of symptoms, but of syndromes as well.

References

1 Arbeitsgemeinschaft für Methodik und Dokumentation in der Psychiatrie: Manual; 2. Aufl., 1972; 3. Aufl., 1979 (Springer, Berlin 1972/1979).
2 Angst, J.; Dittrich, A.; Woggon, B.: Reproduzierbarkeit der Faktorenstruktur des AMP-Systems. Int. Pharmacopsychiat. *14:* 319–324 (1979).
3 Baumann, U.: Diagnostische Differenzierungsfähigkeit von Psychopathologie-Skalen. Arch. Psychiat. Nerv. Krankh. *219:* 89–103 (1974).
4 Baumann, U.: Unveröffentlichtes Manuskript (1974).
5 Baumann, U.; Angst, J.: Methodological development of the AMP system; in Boissier, Neuropsychopharmacology, vol. 9, pp. 72–78 (Excerpta Medica, Amsterdam 1975).
6 Baumann, U.; Woggon, B.: Interrater-Reliabilität bei Diagnosen, AMP-Syndromen und AMP-Symptomen. Arch. Psychiat. Nerv. Krankh. *227:* 3–15 (1979).
7 Cranach, M. v.; Hippius, H.; Wegscheider, R.: A factor analytic study of depressive symptomatology; in Garattini, Depressive disorders, pp. 203–210 (Schattauer, Stuttgart 1978).
8 Gebhardt, R.; Pietzcker, A.; Freudenthal, K.; Langer, C.: Die Bildung von Syndromen im AMP-System Arch. Psychiat. NervKrankh. *231:* 93–110 (1981).
9 Hentschel, U.; Schubö, W.; Zerssen, D. v.: Diagnostische Klassifikationsversuche mit zwei standardisierten psychiatrischen Schätzskalen. Arch. Psychiat. Nerv. Krankh. *221:* 283–301 (1976).
10 Lienert, G. A.: Testaufbau und Testanalyse (Beltz, Weinheim 1969).
11 Maxwell, A. E.: Difficulties in a dimensional description of symptomatology. Br. J. Psychiat. *121:* 19–26 (1972).
12 Maurer-Groeli, Y. A.: Untersuchung zur Interraterreliabilität des AMP-Systems. Arch. Psychiat. Nerv. Krankh. *221:* 321–329 (1976).
13 Mombour, W.; Gammel, G.; Zerssen, D. v.; Heyse, H.: Die Objektivierung psychiatrischer Syndrome durch multifaktorielle Analyse des psychopathologischen Befundes. Nervenarzt *44:* 352–358 (1973).
14 Pietzcker, A.; Gebhardt, R.; Freudenthal, K.; Langer, C.: Korrelationsstatistischer Vergleich der verschiedenen Faktorenanalysen des AMP-Systems. Arch. Psychiat. Nerv. Krankh. *231:* 259–268 (1982).
15 Sulz-Blume, B.; Sulz, K.-D.; Cranach, M. v.: Zur Stabilität der Faktorenstruktur der AMDP-Skalen. Arch. Psychiat. Nerv. Krankh. *227:* 353–366 (1979).
16 Tegeler, J.; Lehmann, E.; Quadbeck, H.: Teststatistischer Vergleich von Fremdbeurteilungs- (AMP) und Selbstbeurteilungs-Verfahren (EWL-K) bei schizophrenen Patienten. Arzneimittel-Forsch. *30:* 1210 (1980).
17 Wegscheider, R.: Empirische Diagnostik aufgrund klinischer Schätzskalen; unveröffentlichte Diplomarbeit, München (1977).
18 Woggon, B.: Untersuchung zum Einfluss von Diagnose und Hospitalisierungs-

dauer auf die Retest-Reliabilität des psychopathologischen Erstbefundes (AMP-System). Int. Pharmacopsychiat. *14:* 228–242 (1979).
19 Woggon, B.: AMP-Syndrom-Interkorrelationen (1981 in Vorbereitung).
20 Woggon, B.; Dittrich, A.: Konstruktion übergeordneter AMP-Skalen: 'manisch-depressives' und 'schizophrenes' Syndrom. Int. Pharmacopsychiat. *14:* 325–337 (1979).
21 Woggon, B.; Dittrich, A.; Luckner, N. v.; Keller, W.: Untersuchung zur Stabilität der faktoriellen Struktur des AMP-Systems im Behandlungsverlauf (1981 in Vorbereitung).
22 Woggon, B.; Jau, B.; Meyer, H.; Schnyder, B.; Storck, U.; Täuber, M.: Untersuchung zur Retest-Reliabilität des psychophatologischen Erstbefundes (AMP-System). Int. Pharmacopsychiat. *14:* 245–259 (1979).
23 Zerssen, D. v.: Syndrom; in Müller, Lexikon der Psychiatrie, p. 508 (Springer, Berlin 1973).
24 AMDP. Empirische Befunde zur Psychopathologie. AMDP-Testmanual (Springer, Berlin 1983).

Prof. Dr. phil. U. Baumann, Institut für Psychologie der Universität, Akademiestrasse 22, A-5020 Salzburg (Austria)

Mod. Probl. Pharmacopsychiat., vol. 20, pp. 88–99 (Karger, Basel 1983)

The Syndrome Scales in the AMDP-System

A. Pietzcker[a], *R. Gebhardt*[a], *A. Strauss*[b], *M. Stöckel*[a], *C. Langer*[a]
K. Freudenthal[a]

[a] Department of Psychiatry, Free University of Berlin, Berlin FRG;
[b] Department of Psychiatry, University of Munich, Munich, FRG

Introduction

There are five different syndrome solutions in the Association for Methodology and Documentation in Psychiatry (AMP) system. Their descriptions are summarized by *Baumann* et al. [this volume]. In that chapter general problems of constructing syndromes are discussed.

In order to obtain final AMDP Scales right after the revision of the AMP-System into the AMDP-System in 1979, it was decided to combine data from the Psychiatric Clinic of the University in Munich with data of the Psychiatric Clinic of the University in Berlin. In this way, a sufficient number of patients was available for the data analysis. Further, it was possible to define them sufficiently sample-independently and to cross-validate them.

Method

Samples

Both centers use the AMDP-System for routine documentation of the psychopathological and somatic symptoms of all patients on admission. Our data analysis is based on symptoms of 2,313 patients through the year 1980 from both centers (1,654 patients from Munich and 659 patients from Berlin). There are differences in distribution of sex, age, and diagnoses between both samples: refer to *Gebhardt* et al. [1983, in prep.] for demographic details and results which cannot be given here. There are 45.6% males in the whole sample. The mean value of age of all the patients is $\bar{x} = 40.2$ years. Males ($\bar{x} = 34.7$ years) are obviously younger than females ($\bar{x} = 43.4$ years).

Diagnostic composition of the sample: organic psychoses (ICD-No. 290–294) 7.5%; schizophrenia (ICD-No. 295) 32.8%;affective psychoses (ICD-Nr. 296) 20.5%; neuroses (ICD No. 300) 15.4%; alcohol and drug dependence (ICD No. 303–305) 6.4%; all other diagnoses 17.4%.

Method of Scale Construction

All the 140 AMDP items of psychopathological and somatic data except 'menstrual disturbances' are included in the analysis. The items are scaled 0 = not present, 1 = mild, 2 = moderate, 3 = severe.

Main components analyses with 1 in the diagonal are calculated as factor extraction methods by means of the BMDP programs [*Dixon,* 1979]. The subsequent rotation is made with the orthogonal Varimax method. In the Berlin sample and separately in the Munich sample factor analyses are computed with the extraction of 12, 11, 10, 9, and 8 factors. For further crossvalidation the Munich sample as well as the Berlin sample are rondomized in split-halfs. By this procedure, a total of 30 factor analyses was carried out.

A symptom is selected as marker item for a syndrome only if it is possible to associate it unequivocally with a factor in the majority of the 30 factor analyses. For this selection factor loadings of $a \geqq 0.35$ are required as well as the specifity for the factor according to the criterion $a^2/h^2 \geqq 0.50$ [*Fürntratt,* 1969]. Subsequently, item analyses are computed by means of special SPSS programs [*Nie* et al., 1979].

Results

Altogether 70 items are associated with the syndromes, which are factor analyzed once again as a reduced item pool. According to the method of *Fischer and Roppert* [1964], a comparison of factor structure between the Munich solution and the Berlin solution is conducted. An extremely high similarity of the results of the factor analyses of both samples is found. The similarity S between both factor matrices reached a value of S = 0.989. The similarities of the individual factors lie between S = 0.87 and S = 0.97. A value of $S \geqq 0.80$ is regarded as a measure of high similarity.

Table I. Paranoid-hallucinatory syndrome (PARHAL)

AMDP item	P	r_{it}	a	h^2	a^2/h^2
Delusional mood	19	0.67	0.74	0.58	0.94
Delusional perceptions	12	0.65	0.73	0.53	1.00
Sudden delusional idea	8	0.48	0.55	0.33	0.92
Delusional ideas	17	0.60	0.67	0.48	0.94
Systematized delusions	10	0.54	0.63	0.41	0.97
Delusional dynamics	15	0.67	0.73	0.57	0.93
Delusions of reference	15	0.59	0.68	0.48	0.96
Delusions of persecution	19	0.60	0.68	0.50	0.92
Verbal hallucinations	13	0.39	0.46	0.23	0.92
Bodily hallucinations	5	0.38	0.46	0.22	0.96
Depersonalization	8	0.33	0.41	0.18	0.93
Thought withdrawal	3	0.31	0.39	0.16	0.95
Other feelings of alien influence	7	0.45	0.53	0.29	0.97

P = Percentage of occurrence; r_{it} = item-test correlation (part-whole corrected); a = factor loading; h^2 = communality; a^2/h^2 = specificity of the item for the factor. Statistics of the syndrome: mean value $\bar{x}$ = 2.89; standard deviation s = 5.18; skewness = 2.10; kurtosis = 4.17; reliability r_{tt} = 0.86; percentage of the extracted variance explained by the factor: VA % = 18.5

Table II. Depressive syndrome (DEPRES)

AMDP item	P	r_{it}	a	h^2	a^2/h^2
Rumination	21	0.41	0.42	0.34	0.52
Feeling of loss of feeling	9	0.39	0.45	0.29	0.70
Felt loss of vitality	32	0.59	0.62	0.49	0.78
Depressed mood	58	0.60	0.62	0.55	0.70
Hopelessness	32	0.54	0.59	0.45	0.77
Feelings of inadequacy	31	0.51	0.55	0.43	0.70
Feelings of guilt	15	0.42	0.49	0.33	0.73
Inhibition of drive	16	0.29	0.36	0.28	0.46
Worse in the morning	13	0.40	0.48	0.27	0.85
Interrupted sleep	57	0.45	0.60	0.46	0.78
Shortened sleep	38	0.38	0.57	0.44	0.74
Early waking	18	0.44	0.56	0.36	0.87
Decreased appetite	44	0.44	0.51	0.34	0.77

Statistics of the syndrome: $\bar{x}$ = 7.44; s = 6.64; skewness = 1.14; kurtosis = 1.00; r_{tt} = 0.81; VA % = 14.7.

Table III. Psychoorganic syndrome (PSYORG)

AMDP item	P	r_{it}	a	h^2	a^2/h^2
Clouded consciousness	3	0.24	0.35	0.13	0.94
Disturbances of orientation:					
Time	9	0.68	0.83	0.69	1.00
Place	6	0.69	0.86	0.75	0.99
Situation	6	0.60	0.81	0.66	0.99
Self	2	0.42	0.61	0.39	0.95
Disturbances of					
Apperception	25	0.47	0.50	0.41	0.61
Memorization	26	0.52	0.51	0.44	0.59
Retention	19	0.48	0.50	0.42	0.60
Confabulation	3	0.39	0.48	0.26	0.89
Lack of self-care	7	0.36	0.48	0.26	0.87

Statistics of the syndrome: $\bar{x}$ = 1.77; s = 3.22; skewness = 3.24; kurtosis = 13.40; r_{tt} = 0.79; VA % = 14.6.

Table IV. Manic syndrome (MANI)

AMDP item	P	r_{it}	a	h^2	a^2/h^2
Flight of ideas	11	0.56	0.69	0.52	0.92
Euphoria	11	0.62	0.74	0.58	0.94
Exaggerated self-esteem	7	0.43	0.56	0.34	0.92
Increased drive	20	0.66	0.72	0.59	0.88
Motor restlessness	32	0.43	0.51	0.39	0.67
Logorrhea	10	0.44	0.60	0.37	0.97
Excessive social contact	8	0.45	0.52	0.35	0.77

Statistics of the syndrome: $\bar{x}$ = 1.82; s = 3.12; skewness = 2.55; kurtosis = 7.27; r_{tt} = 0.78; VA % = 12.9.

Eight syndromes could be extracted from the different factor analyses: paranoid-hallucinatory, depressive, psychoorganic, manic, hostility, autonomic, apathy, and obsessive-compulsive (table I-VIII). A neurological syndrome was only constituted by 4 items; in the patients' findings on admission neurological signs can rarely be found but neurological signs are needed for description of side effects in the course of psychopharmacological treatment. For this reason a neurological ad hoc syndrome (table IX) was defined on the basis of clinical considerations

Table V. Hostility syndrome (HOST)

AMDP item	P	r_{it}	a	h^2	a^2/h^2
Suspiciousness	22	0.28	0.39	0.27	0.56
Dysphoria	21	0.41	0.61	0.39	0.95
Irritability	21	0.53	0.66	0.51	0.85
Aggressiveness	15	0.46	0.61	0.43	0.87
Lack of feeling ill	21	0.56	0.58	0.48	0.70
Lack of insight	29	0.58	0.63	0.52	0.76
Uncooperativeness	14	0.51	0.66	0.46	0.95

Statistics of the syndrome: $\bar{x} = 2.72$; s = 3.71; skewness = 1.69; kurtosis = 2.69; r_{tt} = 0.75; VA % = 10.8.

Table VI. Autonomic syndrome (AUTON)

AMDP item	P	r_{it}	a	h^2	a^2/h^2
Hypochondriasis	9	0.24	0.38	0.18	0.80
Nausea	9	0.35	0.51	0.29	0.90
Breathing difficulties	7	0.29	0.46	0.22	0.96
Dizziness	13	0.39	0.58	0.34	0.99
Palpitations	13	0.44	0.59	0.36	0.97
Cardiac Pain	9	0.39	0.51	0.29	0.90
Increased perspiration	19	0.31	0.49	0.27	0.89
Headache	17	0.33	0.45	0.23	0.88
Hot flashes	3	0.29	0.44	0.21	0.92

Statistics of the syndrome: $\bar{x} = 1.62$; s = 2.58; skewness = 2.55; kurtosis = 8.82; r_{tt} = 0.65; VA % = 9.8.

Table VII. Apathy syndrome (APA)

AMDP item	P	r_{it}	a	h^2	a^2/h^2
Inhibited thinking	13	0.40	0.55	0.38	0.80
Retarded thinking	29	0.52	0.66	0.49	0.89
Circumstantial thinking	24	0.22	0.47	0.36	0.61
Restricted thinking	34	0.34	0.55	0.40	0.76
Blunted affect	20	0.42	0.54	0.34	0.86
Affective rigidity	17	0.39	0.47	0.29	0.76
Lack of drive	38	0.45	0.49	0.37	0.65
Social withdrawal	44	0.37	0.37	0.30	0.46

Statistics of the syndrome: $\bar{x} = 3.88$; s = 3.86; skewness = 1.30; kurtosis = 1.79; r_{tt} = 0.69; VA % = 11.3.

Table VIII. Obsessive-compulsive syndrome (OBSESS)

AMDP item	P	r_{it}	a	h^2	a^2/h^2
Obsessive thoughts	5	0.50	0.75	0.57	0.99
Compulsive impulses	2	0.58	0.79	0.62	1.00
Compulsive actions	2	0.50	0.75	0.56	1.00

Statistics of the syndrome: $\bar{x} = 0.16$; $s = 0.76$; skewness = 6.77; kurtosis = 55.69; $r_{tt} = 0.69$; VA % = 7.4.

Table IX. Neurological syndrome (the neurological syndrome is an 'ad hoc' syndrome, built on the basis of clinical considerations, not of factor analysis)

	Scaling
Hypertonia Hypotonia Tremor Dyskinesia Hypokinesia Akathisia Ataxia Nystagmus	0 = absent 1 = mild 2 = moderate 3 = severe
Convulsions	0 = absent 3 = present

at the AMDP Meeting in Zürich, October 1982. No statistics of this syndrome are calculated, because the admission data are inappropriate.

Table I-VIII show the parameters and the statistics of the syndromes of the factor analyses carried out in the total sample (n = 2,313) and the pool of the 70 items chosen as marker-items for the syndromes.

For the individual items, the tables include the percentage of occurrence (P) of each item in the total sample; the item-test correlations r_{it}, which are part-whole corrected because the item is a part of the syndrome; the factor loadings a, the communalities h^2 and the coefficients a^2/h^2. The coefficient a^2/h^2 is a measure of the specificity of the association of the item to the factor [*Fürntratt,* 1969].

The mean value, $\bar{x}$, and the standard deviation, s, the skewness and the kurtosis of the score distributions are given in the statistics of the syndrome. The reliability, r_{tt}, is a measure of internal consistency [*Cronbach,*

Table X. Transformation of raw scores into T-values (after log transf.)

Raw scores	PARHAL	DEPRES	PSYORG	MANI	HOST	AUTON	APA
0	43	31	42	42	40	42	35
1	50	38	51	51	48	51	43
2	54	43	56	56	52	56	48
3	56	46	60	59	56	60	52
4	59	48	62	62	58	63	54
5	60	50	65	64	60	65	56
6	62	52	67	66	62	67	58
7	63	53	68	68	63	69	60
8	64	55	70	69	65	71	61
9	65	56	71	71	66	72	62
10	66	57	72	72	67	73	63
11	67	58	73	73	68	74	64
12	68	59	74	74	69	75	65
13	69	59	75	75	69	76	66
14	69	60	76	76	70	77	67
15	70	61	77	76	71	78	68
16	70	61	78	77	72	79	69
17	71	62	79	78	72	80	69
18	72	63	79	79	73	81	70
19	72	63	80	79	73	81	70
20	73	64	81	80	74	82	71
21	73	64	81		74		72
				max	max		
22	73	65	82				72
23	74	65	82				73
24	74	66	83				
							max
25	75	66	83				
26	75	66					
27	75	67					
						max	
28	75	67					
29	76	67					
30	76	68					
			max				
31	76	68					
32	76	68					
33	77	69					
34	77	69					
35		69					
.							
.							
39							
	max	max					

1966]. The percentage of the extracted variance explained by the factor is indicated by VA%.

In order to make comparable the syndromes constituted by different item numbers, the raw scores are transformed into T-values ($\bar{x} = 50$, $s = 10$). The score distributions are negatively skewed, therefore this T transformation was preceded by logarithmic transformation. The T-values of each syndrome from the raw scores can be directly read from table X. For the obsessive-compulsive syndrome, no T-transformation was calculated, because it only consists of 3 items.

A detailed but still accessible description of psychopathology can be made by means of the eight first-order syndromes. For some selected problems it could be sufficient to deal with a less detailed description of the psychopathological findings on fewer dimensions. Therefore, second-order factors corresponding to the procedure of other authors [*Baumann* et al., this volume], are computed. Only 2 or 3 factors were extracted from the 70 items associated with the eight first-order factors. A stable factor structure with three factors results from factor analyses of the various samples: the psychotic factor (table XI), the depressive factor (table XII) and the psychoorganic factor (table XIII). The first two factors are largely similar to the second-order factors of the AMP-System. The third second-order factor is arising for the first time. It could not appear in the corresponding analyses in the AMP-System because of the item selection and sample selection.

The similarity is high between the syndrome scales of the AMDP-System and the five syndrome solutions which were formed within different samples in the AMP-System: 60 (86%) of the 70 marker items of the AMDP syndromes are associated with the corresponding syndromes of all different AMP syndrome solutions or most ot them; 5 of the remaining 10 marker items are newly introducted into the AMDP-System (table XIV). Therefore, they could not be integrated in the corresponding syndromes of the AMP-System.

A stuporous (catatonic) factor was extracted in most of the solutions of the AMP-System. In the AMDP-System, a corresponding factor could not be extracted. The main reason for this is that many items which constituted the stuporous syndrome in the AMP-System were not included in the AMDP-System.

Finally, an example of the comparability of the AMDP syndrome scales with the AMP syndrome scales is given here. A first hint to the validity of the syndrome scales is given by the fact that clinical groups can

Table XI. First second-order syndrome (psychotic syndrome)

AMDP item	Syndrome	a	h^2	a^2/h^2	r_{it}
Delusional mood	PARHAL	0.73	0.53	1.00	0.65
Delusional dynamics	PARHAL	0.72	0.53	0.98	0.66
Delusional ideas	PARHAL	0.68	0.45	1.00	0.60
Delusional perceptions	PARHAL	0.67	0.46	0.98	0.61
Delusions of reference	PARHAL	0.66	0.43	1.00	0.57
Delusions of persecution	PARHAL	0.65	0.43	0.98	0.58
Systematized delusions	PARHAL	0.60	0.37	0.97	0.55
Sudden delusional idea	PARHAL	0.54	0.30	0.97	0.47
Other feelings of alien influence	PARHAL	0.50	0.26	0.96	0.43
Lack of insight	HOST	0.46	0.31	0.68	0.41
Lack of feeling ill	HOST	0.43	0.32	0.58	0.40
Verbal hallucinations	PARHAL	0.42	0.18	0.98	0.37
Bodily hallucinations	PARHAL	0.41	0.17	0.99	0.36
Depersonalization	PARHAL	0.40	0.16	1.0	0.32
Thought withdrawal	PARHAL	0.36	0.13	1.0	0.30

Statistics of the syndrome: $\bar{x} = 3.99$; s = 6.06; skewness = 1.89; kurtosis = 3.39; r_{tt} = 0.85; VA % = 36.4

Table XII. Second second-order syndrome (depressive syndrome)

AMDP item	Syndrome	a	h^2	a^2/h^2	r_{it}
Depressed mood	DEPRES	0.65	0.49	0.86	0.62
Felt loss of vitality	DEPRES	0.60	0.38	0.95	0.55
Hopelessness	DEPRES	0.58	0.36	0.93	0.55
Feelings of inadequacy	DEPRES	0.54	0.33	0.88	0.50
Lack of drive	APA	0.52	0.27	1.00	0.42
Rumination	DEPRES	0.52	0.28	0.97	0.44
Retarded thinking	APA	0.47	0.30	0.74	0.37
Feelings of guilt	DEPRES	0.47	0.22	1.00	0.42
Feeling of loss of feeling	DEPRES	0.46	0.21	1.00	0.39
Decreased appetite	DEPRES	0.45	0.22	0.92	0.39
Social withdrawal	APA	0.45	0.22	0.92	0.36
Inhibited thinking	APA	0.44	0.24	0.81	0.34
Inhibition of drive	DEPRES	0.43	0.19	0.97	0.37
Worse in the morning	DEPRES	0.40	0.19	0.84	0.36
Restricted thinking	APA	0.36	0.23	0.56	0.26
Interrupted sleep	DEPRES	0.36	0.15	0.86	0.26

Statistics of the syndrome: $\bar{x} = 9.14$; s = 7.46; skewness = 1.11; kurtosis = 1.19; VA% = 35.7; r_{tt} = 0.81

Table XIII. Third second-order syndrome (psychoorganic syndrome)

AMDP item	a	h^2	a^2/h^2	r_{it}
Disturbances of orientation:				
Place	0.78	0.61	1.00	0.68
Time	0.76	0.57	1.00	0.68
Situation	0.73	0.54	0.99	0.60
Disturbances of:				
Apperception	0.58	0.37	0.91	0.47
Memorization	0.58	0.37	0.91	0.52
Retention	0.55	0.33	0.92	0.48
Orientation: self	0.53	0.29	0.97	0.42
Confabulation	0.49	0.24	1.00	0.39
Lack of self-care	0.47	0.22	1.00	0.36
Clouded Consciousness	0.31	0.10	0.96	0.24

Statistics of the syndrome: $\bar{x} = 1.77$; $s = 3.22$; skewness = 3.24; kurtosis = 13.40; VA% = 27.8; $r_{tt} = 0.81$

Table XIV. Item concordance between the AMDP scales and the corresponding AMP syndromes (in parentheses are given the number of items which are newly included in the AMDP-System; they therefore could not be marker-items in an AMDP syndrome)

AMDP syndrome scale	Item number K	Identical choice of x items as marker-items in			
		all five x	four x	three x	AMP syndrome solutions
PARHAL	13 (1)	11	–	–	[*Baumann* et al., this volume]
DEPRES	13 (3)	4	2	2	
PSYORG	10 (1)	6	–	2	
MANI	7	6	1	–	
HOST	7	5	2	–	
AUTON	9	7	–	2	
APA	8	2	3	2	
OBSESS	3	3	–	–	

be discriminated by their means [*Gebhardt* et al., in prep.]. If the syndrome profiles of the clinical groups as they are represented in the AMP syndrome scales [*Gebhardt* et al., 1981] are compared to their representation by means of the syndrome scales of the AMDP-System [*Gebhardt* et al., 1983], the high similarity in the syndrome profiles is evident.

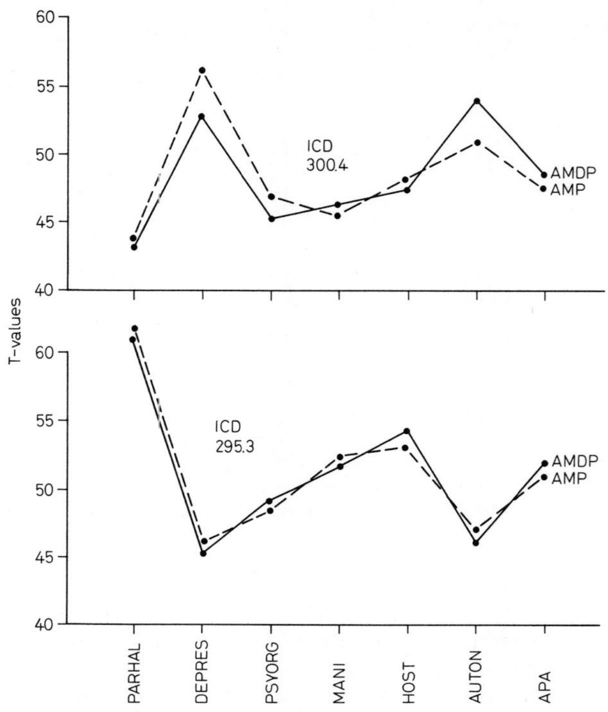

Fig. 1. Comparison between the syndrome profiles of neurotic depressives (ICD No. 300.4, n = 364 AMP Berlin versus n = 207 AMDP Berlin and Munich) and paranoid schizophrenics (ICD No. 295.3, n = 404 AMP Berlin versus n = 354 AMDP Berlin and Munich).

Figure 1 shows the syndrome profiles of paranoid-hallucinatory schizophrenia (ICD No. 295.3) and depressive neurosis (ICD No. 300.4). The syndrome profile of paranoid-hallucinatory schizophrenia is represented in the scales of the AMP-System for a group of n = 404 patients from Berlin through the years 1971–1976, and in the scales of the AMDP-System for 354 patients from Berlin and Munich through the year 1980. The syndrome profiles of the depressive neurosis are represented in the scales of the AMP System for n = 364 patients from Berlin through the years 1971 to 1976, and in the scales of the AMDP-System for n = 207 patients from Berlin and Munich through the year 1980.

Conclusions

Factor analyses based on data from Munich and Berlin (n = 2,313 patients) resulted in stable, reliable, and sample-independent syndrome scales. In spite of the differences between the Munich sample and the Berlin sample, identical syndromes in both patient samples are found. The syndrome scales satisfy test statistical criteria. It seems justifiable to use the syndrome scales for the description of psychopathology (and partly of the somatic findings, too) in scientific evaluations. Because of the favorable similarity with the syndromes in the AMP-System, there is a good comparability between new studies based on AMDP syndrome scales and the already published scientific work using the former AMP Scales.

References

Cronbach, L. J.: Essentials of psychologic testing (Harper & Row, New York 1966).

Dixon, W. J.; Brown, M.B.: Biomedical Computer Programs, P-Series (University of California Press, Berkeley 1979).

Fischer, G.; Roppert, J.: Bemerkungen zu einem Verfahren der Transformationsanalyse. Arch. ges. Psychol. *116:* 98–100 (1964).

Fürntratt, E.: Zur Bestimmung der Anzahl interpretierbarer gemeinsamer Faktoren in Faktorenanalysen psychologischer Daten. Diagnostica *15:* 62–75 (1969).

Gebhardt, R.; Pietzcker, A.; Freudenthal, K.; Langer, C.: Die Bildung von Syndromen im AMP-System. Arch. Psychiat. Nerv. Krankh. *231:* 93–109 (1981).

Gebhardt, R.; Pietzcker, A.; Strauss, A.; Stöckel, M.; Langer, C.; Freudenthal, K.: Skalenbildung im AMDP-System. Arch. Psychiat. Nerv. Krankh. (in press, 1983).

Gebhardt, R.; Pietzcker, A.; Stöckel, M.; Langer, C.; Freudenthal, K.: Diagnostische Differenzierungsfähigkeit der AMDP-Syndromprofile (in preparation).

Nie, N. H.; Hull, H.; Jenkins, J. G.; Steinbrinner, K.; Bent, D. H.: SPSS. Statistical package for the social sciences (McGraw Hill, New York 1979).

A. Pietzcker, MD, Department of Psychiatry, Free University of Berlin,
Eschenallee 3, D-1000 Berlin 19 (FRG)

Mod. Probl. Pharmacopsychiat., vol. 20, pp. 100–106 (Karger, Basel 1983)

Comparison between AMDP and EWL-K Ratings in Schizophrenic Patients

J. Tegeler, E. Lehmann, H. Quadbeck

Department of Psychiatry, University of Düsseldorf, Düsseldorf, FRG

Introduction

It has become common practice to utilize multiple psychological measurements like rating scales and symptom checklists to assess the multidimensional aspects of clinical symptoms and patients' behaviour. Although considerable research has been conducted on the reliability and factorial structure of the Association for Methodology and Documentation in Psychiatry (AMDP) system, little attention has been paid to concordances and discordances between observer ratings and self-reports. *Maurer and Dittrich* [1979] published a comparison of the AMDP-System and a self-report questionnaire, APZ. For acute schizophrenic patients the degree of psychopathology correlated negatively with the testability. When the patients were symptomatically improved, this correlation could not be detected anymore. *Debus* [1974] found in his sample of schizophrenic and depressive patients high correlations between self-report ratings (EWL-K) and psychiatrist's ratings (BSK).

The EWL-K [*Janke and Debus,* 1974] is an adjective checklist which consists of 124 items. The subjects were asked to decide whether the adjective corresponds to his present emotional state or not. This schedule is not intended for acute psychotic patients, but experience has shown that after improvement schizophrenic and depressive patients are able to respond accurately to this checklist. The EWL-K is sensitive and reliable to evaluate changes of emotional states in volunteers [*Janke and Debus,* 1972; *Lehmann and Hopes,* 1977] and in schizophrenic and depressive patients [*Gebhardt,* 1972; *Debus,* 1974].

In our study we were interested in the following questions: (1) Are there essential differences in reliability between AMDP and EWL-K ratings in schizophrenic patients? (2) Are there essential concordances or discordances between the AMDP and EWL-K ratings?

Methods

Sample

The sample consisted of 106 women and 46 men with a mean age of 40,3 years (range 20–46 years) and a mean duration of illness of 8,4 years; 101 patients had a paranoid-hallucinatory psychosis (ICD No. 295.3), 35 patients had a chronic schizophrenia (ICD No. 295.6) and 16 patients had a hebephrenia (ICD No. 295.1). All these inpatients were treated with different long-acting neuroleptics in controlled trials. The ratings of the AMDP Psychopathological Scale and of the EWL-K before admission to the trial were included in the study.

Variables

For statistical analysis the scores of the 9 AMDP syndromes based on the factor analysis of *Baumann* [1974] and the scores of the 14 EWL-K factors [*Janke and Debus,* 1974] were used.

Statistics

Part/whole corrected item scale correlations and internal consistencies (Cronbach's alpha) were calculated for the AMDP and EWL-K factors. To describe the correlations between the factors of both scales, Pearson coefficients were performed. In a next step AMDP and EWL-K factors were compared with each other by computation of a combined factor analysis of both scales to prove their correlation and by separate factor analyses of each scale in order to form factors of second rank. The method of principal factoring with iterations was used. The minimum eigenvalue was 1.0. The extraction was followed by a Varimax rotation.

Results

Part/Whole Correlations and Internal Consistencies

Part/whole correlations and internal consistencies of the AMDP-Scales are presented on table I. The alpha coefficients range from 0.55 to 0.79.

Table I. Part/whole correlations and internal consistencies of AMDP Scales

Syndromes	Part/whole correlations		
	range	$\bar{x}$	alpha
Apathy	0.01–0.68	0.49	0.79
Hallucinatory	0.06–0.67	0.43	0.78
Hostility	0.17–0.62	0.44	0.78
Paranoid	0.14–0.68	0.45	0.79
Manic	0.12–0.56	0.43	0.72
Retarded-depressive	0.17–0.66	0.42	0.67
Hypochondriasis	0.08–0.47	0.40	0.57
Catatonic	0.00–0.52	0.25	0.56
Psycho-organic	0.04–0.58	0.25	0.55

Table II. Part/whole correlations and internal consistencies of EWL-K Scales

Scales	Part/whole correlations		
	range	$\bar{x}$	alpha
Activation	0.22–0.68	0.51	0.82
Desactivation	0.33–0.64	0.50	0.83
Tiredness	0.27–0.58	0.49	0.74
Confusion	0.31–0.44	0.47	0.62
Extraversion	0.25–0.53	0.46	0.70
Introversion	0.44–0.62	0.48	0.82
Dreamy state	0.36–0.49	0.48	0.69
Emotional excitement	0.20–0.63	0.47	0.84
Vulnerability	0.36–0.60	0.47	0.73
Self-confidence	0.30–0.48	0.47	0.70
Anxiety	0.53–0.64	0.48	0.83
Depression	0.44–0.67	0.50	0.90
Elation	0.46–0.75	0.51	0.88
Aggression	0.28–0.33	0.50	0.62

Table II shows the part/whole correlations and internal consistencies of the EWL-K scales with a range from 0.62 to 0.90.

Correlations of AMDP and EWL-K Factors

Pearson coefficients of the AMDP and EWL-K factors are not listed here, because they reach only values not higher than 0.38.

Table III. Combined factor analysis of AMDP and EWL-K Scales; factor loadings >.40

EWL-K Scales	Factor				
	1	2	3	4	5
Activation	–	–	0.79	–	–
Desactivation	0.67	–	–	–	–
Tiredness	0.75	–	–	–	–
Confusion	0.65	–	–	–	–
Extraversion	–	–	0.73	–	–
Introversion	0.65	–	–	–	–
Dreamy State	0.58	–	–	–	–
Emotional excitement	0.78	–	–	–	–
Vulnerability	0.62	–	–	–	–
Self-confidence	–	–	0.70	–	–
Anxiety	0.81	–	–	–	–
Depression	0.83	–	–	–	–
Elation	–	–	0.87	–	–
Aggression	0.70	–	–	–	–
AMDP-Scales					
Apathy	–	0.82	–	–	–
Hallucinatory	–	–	–	0.85	–
Hostility	–	–	–	–	0.46
Manic	–	–	–	–	0.72
Paranoid	–	–	–	0.89	–
Catatonic	–	0.73	–	–	–
Retarded-depressive	–	0.75	–	–	–
Hypochondriasis	–	0.73	–	–	–
Psycho-organic	–	0.61	–	–	–

Combined Factor Analysis of AMDP and EWL-K Factors (table III)

Five second-order factors are discovered. Factor 1 and factor 3 represent EWL-K dimensions. In the factors 2, 4 and 5 only AMDP syndromes have high loadings.

Factor Analysis of the AMDP Syndromes (table IV)

In factor 1 the following syndromes have high loadings: apathy, catatonic syndrome, retarded-depressive syndrome, hypochondriasis and psycho-organic syndrome. Factor 2 is constituted by the hallucinatory syndrome and the paranoid syndrome. Factor 3 includes hostility and the manic syndrome.

Table IV. Factor analysis of AMDP syndromes; factor loadings >0.40

Scales	Factor		
	1	2	3
Apathy	0.81	–	–
Hallucinatory	–	0.80	–
Hostility	–	–	0.46
Manic	–	–	0.79
Paranoid	–	0.96	–
Catatonic	0.70	–	–
Retarded-depressive	0.79	–	–
Hypochondriasis	0.76	–	–
Psycho-organic	0.63	–	–

Table V. Factor analysis of EWL-K Scales; factor loadings >0.40

Scales	Factor	
	1	2
Activation	–	0.79
Desactivation	0.68	–
Tiredness	0.75	–
Confusion	0.67	–
Extraversion	–	0.74
Introversion	0.65	–
Dreamy state	0.59	–
Emotional excitement	0.77	–
Vulnerability	0.60	–
Self-confidence	–	0.70
Anxiety	0.82	–
Depression	0.83	–
Elation	–	0.87
Aggression	0.70	–

Factor Analysis of the EWL-K Syndromes (table V)

In factor 1 the following syndromes have high loadings: desactivation, tiredness, confusion, introversion, dreamy state, emotional excitement, vulnerability, anxiety and aggression. Factor 2 includes the syndromes: activation, extraversion, self-confidence and elation.

Discussion

The aim of our study was to test the reliability of AMDP syndromes and EWL-K factors, and whether these scales assess similar or different aspects of clinical symptoms and patient's behaviour.

Levels of internal consistency for the AMDP syndromes apathy, paranoid syndrome, hallucinatory syndrome, hostility and manic syndrome were high (0.71–0.79), whereas alpha coefficients for hypochondriasis, catatonic syndrome and psycho-organic syndrome were only modest (0.55–0.57). *Woggon and Dittrich* [1979] found comparable internal consistency levels for the AMDP syndromes. Results indicate higher levels of internal consistency for the EWL-K factors than for the AMDP factors. *Debus* [1974] published for his sample of schizophrenic and depressive patients comparable Cronbach's alpha coefficients.

Combined and separate factor analyses of the AMDP and EWL-K dimensions identified five factors. For the AMDP-System, factor 1 consists of the syndromes apathy, catatonic syndrome, retarded depressive syndrome, hypochondriasis and psycho-organic syndrome. This factor can be labelled 'schizophrenic residual state'. The hallucinatory and paranoid syndromes have high loadings in factor 2, which can be defined as 'acute schizophrenic state'. Factor 3 includes the hostility and manic syndromes; it can be called 'excitation state'.

For the EWL-K, factor 1 consists of the following dimensions: desactivation, tiredness, confusion, introversion, emotional excitement, vulnerability, anxiety, depression and aggression. This factor can be defined as 'desactivation with negative emotional state'. In factor 2 the dimensions activation, extraversion, self-confidence and elation show high loadings. We call this factor 'activation with positive emotional state'.

We found that the AMDP and EWL-K are reliable instruments to evaluate different dimensions of patient's behaviour. Our results emphasize the importance of using rating scales as well as symptom checklists in clinical research to assess the multidimensional aspects of symptoms and patient's behaviour.

References

Baumann, U.: Diagnostische Differenzierungsfähigkeit von Psychopathologie-Skalen. Arch. psychiat. NervKrankh. *219:* 89–103 (1974).

Debus, G.: Selbst- und Fremdeinstufungen des aktuellen Befindens in psychopharmakologischen Längsschnittuntersuchungen. Arzneimittel-Forsch. *24:* 996–1001 (1974).

Gebhardt, R.: Veränderungen der subjektiven Befindlichkeit psychotischer Patienten unter neuroleptischer Therapie. Pharmakopsychiatr. Neuro-Psychopharmakol. *5:* 295–300 (1972).

Janke, W.; Debus, G.: Double-blind psychometric evaluation of Pimozide and Haloperidol versus placebo in emotionally labile volunteers under two different work load conditions. Pharmakopsychiatr. Neuro-Psychopharmakol. *5:* 34–51 (1972).

Janke, W.; Debus, G.: Eigenschaftswörterliste (Verlag für Psychologie Dr. C. J. Hogrefe, Göttingen 1974).

Lehmann, E.; Hopes, H.: Differential effects of a single dose of Imipramine and Lopramine in healthy subjects varying in their level of depression. Prog. Neuro-Psychopharmacol. *1:* 155–164 (1977).

Maurer, Y.; Dittrich, A.: Vergleich von Selbst- und Fremdbeurteilung bei schizophrenen Patienten. Pharmakopsychiatr. Neuro-Psychopharmakol. *12:* 375–382 (1979).

Woggon, B.; Dittrich, A.: Konstruktion übergeordneter AMP-Skalen: 'manisch-depressives' und 'schizophrenes' Syndrom. Int. Pharmacopsychiat. *14:* 325–337 (1979).

Dr. J. Tegeler, Psychiatrische Klinik der Universität – Rheinische Landesklinik Düsseldorf, Bergische Landstrasse 2, D-4000 Düsseldorf (FRG)

Mod. Probl. Pharmacopsychiat., vol. 20, pp. 107–118 (Karger, Basel 1983)

Classification Analysis of Depression through AMDP-4

M. Paes de Sousa, M. L. Figueira, M. H. Nicolau

Department of Psychiatry, University of Lisbon Medical School, Lisbon, Portugal

When studying depression, *Kraepelin* [1921] differentiated the endogenous or psychotic depressive syndromes from the exogenous, neurotic, psychogenic or reactive ones. This dichotomy has been extremely debated, defended by some, denied by others, and this dilemma has been maintained up to now.

The point of view of *Kraepelin* [1921] was soon challenged by several authors – like for instance *Mapother* [1926], *Lewis* [1934], etc. – who supported the unitary concept of depression, since they did not recognize any clinical distinction between both types of depression.

Since then, there have been many attempts of clinical classification of depressions, some based on a dualist concept, others on a unitary one, classifications which intend to include the variety of clinical pictures described by several authors.

When we analyze the different classifications of depression – from classical or modern authors (international ones, like the ICD-9, or the American ones, like that from the School of St. Louis or the DSM-III) it is evident that they are oriented in two directions: either they underline the depressive heterogeneity which is after all dichotomic (psychotic versus neurotic), or they point out the unity of the depressive syndromes which would have constituted a single disease. Although that dichotomy has been wideley accepted, it is also true that many authors have described intermediate clinical pictures between both depressive poles.

In modern times, with the progress of statistical methods and with their application to psychiatry, the debate between the unitary and the dualist concepts of depression was reopened. There are numerous works applying mathematic procedures to the study of the classification of depressions. An important aspect is the fact that the data analyzed were obtained through questionnaires and rating scales, with or without additional data, which allows the quantification and standardization of the clinical information.

Three multivariate statistical methods have been mainly used: factor analysis, discriminant functions analysis and cluster analysis. The studies of *Hamilton and White* [1959], *Grinker* et al. [1961], *Friedman* et al. [1963], *Kiloh and Garside* [1963], *Carney* et al. [1965], *Mendels and Cochrane* [1968], *Kay* et al. [1969], *Paykel* et al. [1971] and *Kiloh* et al. [1972], using principal components factor analysis, reached some general agreement concerning the polarity between endogenous and neurotic depressions. Also *Kendell* [1968], using discriminant functions analyses, found a separation between neurotic, psychotic and involutional depressive patients, though this distinction was more quantitative than qualitative.

With the use of these types of mathematical techniques, some authors concluded that there is a real separation between the several groups of symptoms – *Carney* et al. [1965], *Sandifer* et al. [1966], *Garside* et al. [1971] and *Andrews* et al. [1973], since the distribution in the factors is bimodal; other authors – *Rosenthal* [1967], *Kendell* [1968], *Kendell and Gourlay* [1970], *Paykel* et al. [1971] and *Kendell and Post* [1973] – describe rather a continuum between neurotic and psychotic, since the distribution is, in their studies, unimodal. *Eysenck* [1970] accepts a 2-dimensional depression, according to his concepts of neuroticism and psychoticism.

In the last years, a more sophisticated technique has been used, the cluster analysis, which already gave classifications of depression, like those of *Overall* et al. [1966] and *Raskin and Crook* [1976], who did not exactly use the cluster analysis, and those of *Pilowsky* et al. [1969], *Paykel* [1971] and *Demel* et al. [1973], in which appears the heterogeneity of depression and the dichotomy psychotic versus neurotic.

Sousa et al. [1976], using the methods of the K-centroids and the *principal components analysis,* found also a distinction between a neurotic and a psychotic group, with an intermediate group, mixed in an axis which separated vital symptoms, present or absent, from anxiety and inhibition. In another study [*Sousa* et al., 1977], made on neurotic and psychotic-depressive patients treated with two different antidepressant drugs, we used the *correspondence analysis.* We found here not only the separation of the two types of depression, but also that of treated and non-treated patients. In a later study, *Sousa* et al. [1980], with the same correspondence analysis, even found a separation between the more and the less severe cases, in an axis of illness severity; this was also nosologic, since the most severe were the psychotic patients and the least severe the neurotic ones.

A controversial problem is that of the involutional depression, also called involutional melancholy, depressive reaction of the involution, depression of late onset or menopausal depression. These different designations represent different conceptions for this clinical picture.

Sousa [1979], in a study performed in elderly patients, found that the most frequent premorbid personalities in the involutional depressions were the cyclothymic and the anankastic ones, the predominant biotype was the pyknic or pyknomorphic, and the most accentuated symptoms were anxiety, agitation, hypochondriacal delusions and obsessive symptoms.

Since a wide discussion has been started concerning involutional depression, we thought that the use of the multivariate statistical techniques – as for instance the correspondence analysis – could be useful in the comparison of endogenous and involutional depressive patients to investigate the existence of a separation between these two groups of depressive patients.

Material and Methods

Our sample is composed of 70 patients suffering from depression, 35 diagnosed as endogenous-depressive patients and 35 as involutional-depressive ones. Among the endogenous, 7 correspond to bipolar depressions and 28 to unipolar depressions.

Table I shows that there is a certain homogeneity between both groups of patients regarding sex, age (although the younger patients are in the endogenous group and the older ones in the involutional group), biotype and personality, though we find a greater number of syntonics within the endogenous-depressive patients and a greater number of anankastics and anxious ones in the involutional-depressive patients; unexpectedly, there is also a larger number of cyclothymics in the involutional-depressive patients, which is in accordance with a previous work already mentioned [*Sousa,* 1979].

We applied our adaptation of the AMDP-4 Psychopathology Scale [*Sousa* et al., in prep.], translated from the German and French revisions [Arbeitsgemeinschaft für Methodik und Dokumentation in der Psychiatrie (AMDP), 1979; *Bobon,* 1981]. This scale comprises 100 items common to all versions, plus 15 items from the French adaptation; these items, rated from 0 to 4 – absent, mild, moderate, severe, very severe – practically cover the whole range of psychopathology. For the present paper, we use the English translation recently published by *Guy and Ban* [1982]; as for the translation of the French items into English for the purpose of the present contribution, it was made by us without the slightest intention of being official.

The fact that we have chosen this measuring instrument was caused not only by the fact that it is the one we use most frequently in the clinical practice of our department, but mainly owing to the circumstance that it is an instrument being more and more used by various researchers, and with a large international use – allowing for cooperative and comparative studies – and also because it transmits the German conceptualization of psychopathology, which is more attached to in Lisbon, as opposed to other measurement instruments like the Mental Status Schedule (MSS) [*Spitzer* et al., 1964], the Present State Examination (PSE) [*Wing* et al., 1974] or the Comprehensive Psychopathological Rating Scale (CPRS) [*Åsberg* et al., 1978].

This scale presents a strong internal consistency and concurrent validation and a high coefficient of interrater reliability, as has been proved by *Sousa* [1982].

The results of the AMDP-4 Scale, with which we have been working, are the results that we obtained from its application to each patient in the first observation and which was done before the start of any therapy whatsoever. The method of data analysis used by us was the correspondence analysis [*Benzecri* et al., 1973]. Of all the items of the scale only 57 items were, in the last analysis, selected, namely the symptoms that came up most frequently. Thus, we had at our disposal, for mathematical analysis, a greater dimensional matrix (70×57), where each line represents an individual described by the scores he respectively obtained in each of the 57 items being considered. Then, a factor analysis of the correspondences was made on the basis of that matrix, the algorithm *Correspo* of Costa Nicolau [*Benzecri* et al., 1973] being used.

We analyzed the first three factors that explain 31% of the total inertia of the system. It is important to point out that the correspondence analysis is similar to a factor analysis. But instead of a Euclidian metric, the Benzecri's analysis uses a χ^2 and keeps a perfect symmetry between the spaces of the subjects and the variables; this is the reason why it is possible to plot the subjects *and* the variables on the same graph.

Table I. Percentages relating to the sex, age, body types and personality of the sample

	Endogenous depression (n=35)	Involutional depression (n=35)
Sex		
Male	28.6	20.0
Female	71.4	80.0
Age, years		
< 40	11.4	–
40–49	20.0	2.9
50–59	51.4	51.4
60–69	8.6	31.4
≥ 70	8.6	14.3
Body types		
Pyknic	57.1	48.6
Leptosomic	42.9	48.6
Athletic	–	2.8
Personality		
Syntonic	40.0	14.3
Cyclothymic	8.6	20.0
Depressive	11.4	11.4
Anankastic	20.0	25.7
Sensitive	17.1	17.1
Anxious	2.9	11.5

Table II. Symptoms which give the highest percentages of contribution to the first factor

Positive side		Negative side	
symptoms	% of contribution	symptoms	% of contribution
Emotional incontinence	6.6	feelings of guilt	1.9
Emotional lability	6.0	perplexity	2.1
Anxious foreboding	2.3	emotional rigidity	2.5
Anxious behavior	3.8	suspiciousness	5.1
Complaintiveness	2.0	delusional ideas	7.9
Inner restlessness	2.4	ambivalence	5.1
Asthenia	2.6	delusions of persecution	11.1
		delusions of reference	8.6
		delusional dynamics	8.4
		systematized delusions	6.8

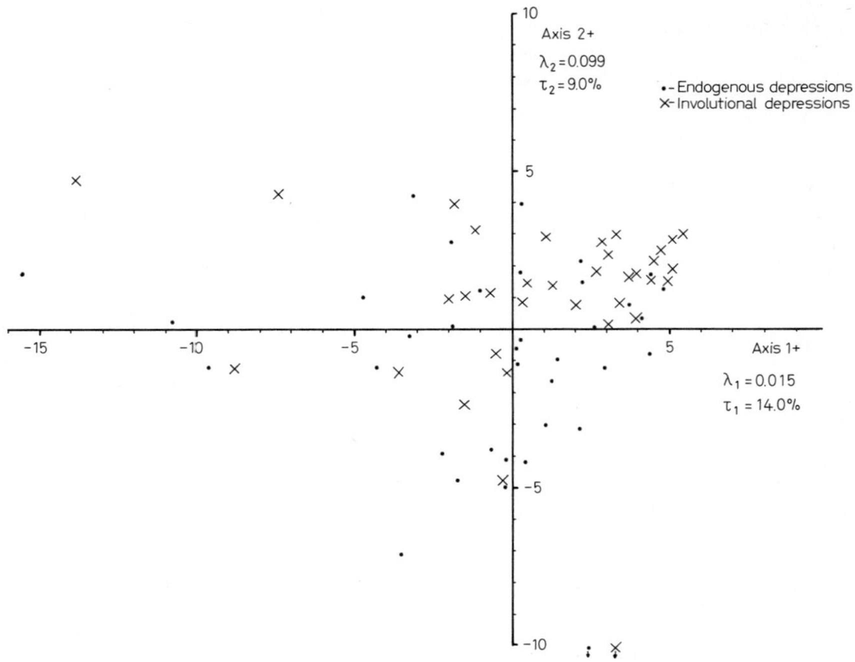

Fig. 1. Factors 1 and 2 (patients).

A final word on the codification problem. When applying the correspondence analysis technique to rating scale data of the AMDP-4 type, it is sometimes useful to adopt one of the two following transformations of data as an alternative to the initial codifications. One may either unfold each variable into two complementary ones, measuring the merit and blame scores; or else one may recode each variable into a number, say k, of presence-absence attributes, by subdividing the measuring scale into K classes, so that the final data matrix submitted to analysis is a 0–1 matrix, which is equivalent to a generalized contingency table. In our case these alternatives were not judged necessary because a hierarchical cluster analysis revealed the same structure of data found in the previous study.

Results and Discussion

The factorial plan 1,2 (fig. 1) explains 23% of the total inertia of the system. The first factor separates patients suffering from great anxiety,

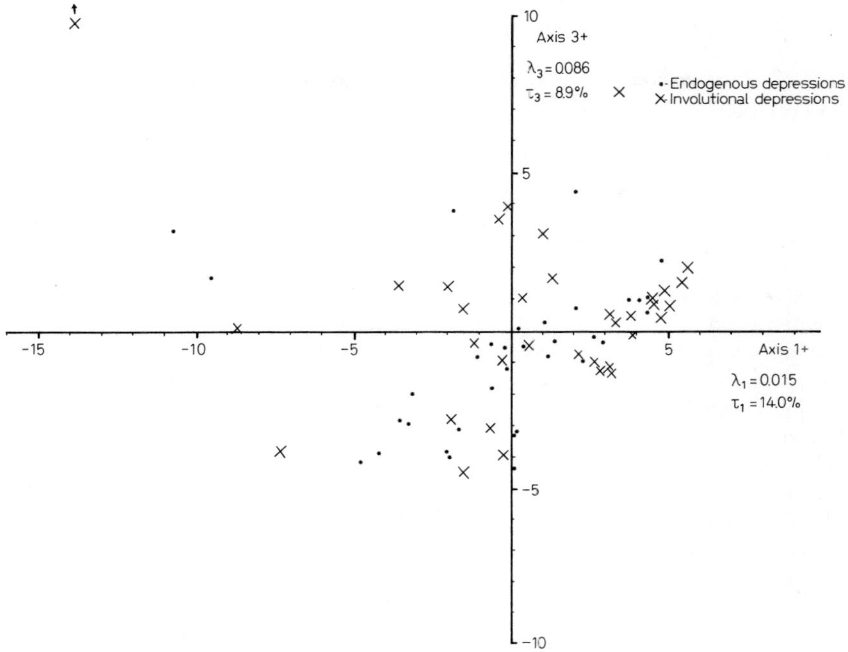

Fig. 2. Factors 1 and 3 (patients).

namely the involutional-depressive ones and some endogenous ones (positive side), from those with delusions who suffer from the two types of depression (negative side).

The symptoms that explain this separation are clearly those of the anxiety sphere (table II). Since anxiety and delusions are at the extreme points of the factorial axis, appearing at opposite sides, it seems that the first factor corresponds to the bipolarization of two symptomatic groups, in a certain way similar to the neurotic and psychotic syndromes, being in a continuum and generally connected respectively with anxious and delusional syndromes.

We may notice a cluster of symptoms in the central part of the axis that are intimately connected to the nuclear depressive syndrome: hopelessness, anxiety, loss of vitality, retardation of thinking, depression, inhibition of drive, lack of drive, feelings of inadequacy, loss of libido, disorder of concentration, uncooperativeness, rumination of thinking, restriction of thinking, suicidal tendencies, disorders of retention, loss of joy of living, feelings of impoverishment, aggressiveness, worse in the morning,

Table III. Symptoms which give the highest percentages of contribution to the second factor

Positive Side		Negative Side	
symptoms	% of contribution	symptoms	% of contribution
Hypochondriacal delusions	2.9	disorder of retention	1.4
Systematized delusions	2.4	loss of joy of living	2.0
Social anxiety	2.0	feelings of guilt	1.6
Blunted affect	4.8	aggressiveness	1.6
Feeling of loss of feeling	4.8	worse in the morning	5.0
Delusions of impoverishment	1.7	irritability	7.1
Anxious foreboding	3.3	disorder of acquisition	3.6
Delusions of persecution	1.7	dysphoria	10.9
Motor restlessness	2.1	better in the afternoon	19.1
Tension	2.8		
Delusional ideas	1.6		
Asthenia	5.5		
Anxious behavior	2.9		

irritability and feelings of guilt. This first factor seems to be a symptomatological one or even syndromatic.

The endogenous and involutional depressive patients are not entirely separated by this axis (fig. 2) and are concentrated in the central area. Both groups of patients have a strong vital symptomatological component as we can verify by the analysis of symptoms that describe them. This first factor is also a factor of intensity or severity of depression; the more severe patients are mainly on the negative side (delusional pole) and the less severe on the positive side (anxious pole). The severity of symptoms is associated with delusions. The involutional depressive patients seem to have a more evident anxious component, probably with neurotic pathoplastic characteristics, than the endogenous depressive ones.

The second factor separates in a more precise way the involutional depressive patients (positive side) from the endogenous (negative side). The symptoms that explain this separation are the anxiety and delusion on the positive side and vital depressive symptoms on the negative side (table III). This factor can be considered as a nosological factor.

Table IV. Symptoms which give the highest percentages of contribution to the third factor

Positive side		Negative side	
symptoms	% of contribution	symptoms	% of contribution
Hypochondriacal delusions	12.4	inhibition of thinking (experienced)	1.9
Better in the afternoon	11.4	aggressiveness	1.8
Worse in the afternoon	6.9	feelings of guilt	2.2
Delusional dynamics	9.2	depersonalization	1.4
Delusions of impoverishment	4.6	suspiciousness	3.0
Ambivalence	1.6	mutism	2.5
Motor restlessness	2.1	blunted affect	2.3
Emotional lability	4.5	feeling of loss of feeling	3.8
Anxious foreboding	1.8	emotional rigidity	9.6
Emotional incontinence	2.5		

The factorial plan 1,3 (fig. 2) explains 23% of the total inertia of the system. In the third factor we have found, on the positive side, symptoms related to agitation and delusions and, on the negative side, vital depressive symptoms (table IV). We have verified that on both sides of the axis, negative and positive, there are involutional and endogenous patients, characterized by different groups of symptoms – on the positive side, delusional, anxious, excitable and emotional labile patients and, one the negative side, marked vital depressive symptoms related to retardation and motor versus affective inhibition.

It is also noticeable that delusions and anxiety separated by the first factor are now clustered in the third factor in opposition to the retardation symptoms. The third factor seems to be a symptomatological factor of inhibition-agitation.

From the fourth factor on, the grouping of symptoms can only be explained on a basis of personality traits. Since the measurement of traits of personality is not included in our description of patients, its appearance is only a subproduct of our analysis. For this reason we decided to stop the analysis at the third factor.

Conclusions

The first conclusion of our research is that from the nosological point of view the two types of depressive patients we studied, involutional and endogenous, have vital depressions and from the symptomatological point of view the involutional depression is characterized by a set of symptoms of the anxious sphere, probably pathoplastic.

In fact, in the first factor, we found a separation between two groups of symptoms: anxious symptoms and delusional symptoms, the first group corresponding to involutional depressive patients and the second to involutional and endogenous depressive patients. This first factor is a symptomatological one and also a severity factor, the depressive patients with anxiety being the less seriously ill and the delusional patients the more seriously ill. This tendency to the separation of groups of symptoms is observable also on the third factor where the symptoms of agitation and inhibition are separated.

Only the second factor seems to be a nosological one, since it separates the depressive involutional patients from the endogenous ones. This separation is due to the anxious symptoms that, although being pathoplastic when present, are sufficiently important to separate the patients in two groups, normally identified as neurotic and psychotic.

The controversy about the concept of involutional depression as an autonomous entity is maintained using only the symptoms as data. It will probably be necessary to use other types of data, for instance the items of other subscales of the AMDP-System.

References

Andrews, G.; Kiloh, L. G.; Neilson, M.: Patterns of depressive illness. Arch. gen. Psychiat. *29:* 670–673 (1973).

Arbeitsgemeinschaft für Methodik und Dokumentation in der Psychiatrie: Das AMDP-System; 3. Aufl. (Springer, Berlin 1979).

Åsberg, M.; Perris, C.; Schalling, D.; Sedvall, G.: The CPRS (a comprehensive psychopathological rating scale) – development and applications of a psychiatric rating scale. Acta psychiat. scand. suppl. 271: 5–27 (1978).

Benzecri, J. P. (ed.): L'analyse des données, vol. 2 (Dunod, Paris 1973).

Bobon, D. P. (ed.): Le système AMDP; 2e éd Coll. Psychol. Sci. hum. (Mardaga, Bruxelles 1981).

Carney, M. H. P.; Roth, M.; Garside, R. F.: Diagnosis of depressive syndromes and prediction of ECT response. Br. J. Psychiat. *111:* 659–674 (1965).

Demel, I.; Gordesch, J.; Katschnig, H.; Pöldinger, W.; Schreiber, V.; Sint, P.: Multivariate procedures in the statistical analysis of psychic and somatic symptoms in depression. Psychother. Psychosom. *22:* 121–130 (1973).

Eysenck, H.J.: The classification of depressive illness. Br. J. Psychiat. *117:* 241–250 (1970).

Friedmann, A.S.; Cowitz, B.; Cohen, H.W.; Branic, K.S.: Syndrome and themes of psychotic depression. A factor analysis. Arch. gen. Psychiat. *9:* 504–509 (1963).

Garside, R.F.; Kay, D.W.K.; Wilson, I.C.; Deathon, I.D.; Roth, M.: Depressive syndromes and the classification of patients. Psychol. Med. *1:* 333–338 (1971).

Grinker, R.R.; Miller, J.; Sabshin, M.; Nunn, R.; Nunnally, J.J.: The phenomena of the depression (Hucker, New York 1961).

Guy, W.; Ban, T.A. (eds): The AMDP-system (Springer, Berlin 1982).

Hamilton, M.; White, J.M.: Clinical syndromes in depressive states. J. ment. Sci. *105:* 985–998 (1959).

Kay, D.W.K.; Garside, R.F.; Beamish, P.; Roy, J.R.: Endogenous and neurotic syndromes of depression: a factor analytic study of 104 cases. Clinical features. Br. J. Psychiat. *115:* 377–388 (1969).

Kendell, R.E.: The classification of depressive illness. Maudsley Monogr. No. 18 (Oxford University Press, London 1968).

Kendell, R.E.; Gourlay, J.: The clinical distinction between psychotic and neurotic depression. Br. J. Psychiat. *117:* 257–260 (1970).

Kendell, R.E.; Post, F.: Depressive illness in late life. Br. J. Psychiat. *122:* 615–617 (1973).

Kiloh, L.G.; Garside, R.F.: The independence of neurotic depression and endogenous depression. Br. J. Psychiat. *109:* 451–463 (1963).

Kiloh, L.G.; Andrews, G.; Neilson, M.; Bianchi, G.N.: The relationship of the syndromes called endogenous and neurotic depression. Br. J. Psychiat. *121:* 183–196 (1972).

Kraepelin, E.: Manic depressive insanity and paranoia; 8th edition translated by Mary Barclay (Churchill-Livingstone, Edinburgh 1921).

Lewis, A.: Melancholia: a clinical survey of depressive states. J. ment. Sci. *80:* 277–378 (1934).

Mapother, E.: Manic depressive psychosis. Br. med. J. *ii:* 872–876 (1926).

Mendels, J.; Cochrane, C.: The nosology of depression: the endogenous-reactive concept. Am. J. Psychiat. *124:* May suppl., 1–11 (1968).

Overall, J.E.; Hollister, L.E.; Johnson, M.; Pennington, V.: Nosology of depression and differential response to drugs. J. Amer. med. Ass. *195:* 946–948 (1966).

Paykel, E.S.: Classification of depressed patients: a cluster analysis derived grouping. Br. J. Psychiat. *118:* 275–288 (1971).

Paykel, E.S.; Prusoff, B.A.; Klerman, G.L.: The endogenous-neurotic continuum in depression: rater independence and factor distributions. J. Psychiat. Res. *8:* 73–90 (1971).

Pilowsky, I.; Levine, S.; Boulton, I.D.M.: The classification of depression by numerical taxonomy. Br. J. Psychiat. *115:* 937–945 (1969).

Raskin, A.; Crook, T.H.: The endogenous-neurotic distinction as a predictor of response to antidepressant drugs. Psychol. Med. *6:* 59–70 (1976).

Rosenthal, S. H.: Neurotic and endogenous depressions: a sceptical view. Br. J. Psychiat. *113:* 1154–1155 (1967).

Sandifer, M. G.; Wilson, I. C.; Green, L.: The two-type thesis of depressive disorders. Am. J. Psychiat. *123:* 93–97 (1966).

Sousa, M. P.: Aspectos psicopatologicos da depressão na 3ª idade. Jornadas de psiquiatria. S João de Deus (Lisboa 1979).

Sousa, M. P.: A traduçao portuguesa do sistema AMDP e problemas afins. Actas Luso-Esp. Neurol. Psiquiatr. *10:* 445–448 (1982).

Sousa, M. P.; Figueira, M. L.; Lopes, J. S.: Contribuição para a classificação em psiquiatria com a utilização do método da taxonomia numérica. Aplicação a um grupo de doentes depressivos. J. Médico XCII (1719): 145–158 (1976).

Sousa, M. P.; Lopes, J. S.; Figueira, M. L.: Nicolau, M. H.; Vieira, C. R.: Utilisation de méthodes d'analyse mathématique taxinomique dans la classification des dépressions (aspects nosologiques et thérapeutiques). Psychol. Med., 13, *13:* 2113–2131 (1981).

Sousa, M. P.; Lopes, J. S.; Figueira, M. L.; Nicolau, M. H.; Vieira, C. R.: Cluster analysis in the study of depressive classification (therapeutic aspects). Acta psiquiat. portug. *26:* 44–61 (1980).

Sousa, M. P. et al. (eds): Draft to the portugese translation of the AMDP system (in preparation).

Spitzer, R. L.; Fleiss, J. L.; Burdock, E. L.; Hardesty, A. S.: The mental status schedule: rationale, reliability and validity. Compreh. Psychiat. *5:* 384–395 (1964).

Wing, J. K.; Cooper, J. E.; Sartorius, N.: Measurement and classification of psychiatric symptoms (Cambridge University Press, London 1974).

M. Paes de Sousa, M.D. Psychiatric Department, Lisbon Medical School, Santa Maria Hospital, 1600 Lisbon (Portugal)

Mod. Probl. Pharmacopsychiat. vol. 20, pp. 119–124 (Karger, Basel 1983)

Rater Training for the Use of Psychiatric Rating Scales:

Recommendations for the AMDP-System

H. Heimann, W. Rein

Department of Psychiatry of the Eberhard-Karls University, Tübingen, FRG

Introduction

The Association for Methodology and Documentation in Psychiatry (AMDP) system [1, 5, 12, 19] includes, besides an anamnestic part which will not be discussed here, rating scales for the evaluation of psychopathological and somatic symptoms. The AMDP-System is therefore not a psychological test in the classical sense [14]. For this reason the competence of the raters, the setting of the rating procedure and the practicability of the scales are of great importance. These basic conditions for the use of the AMDP-System and the possibilities to improve them by rater training will be discussed in this article.

The Problem of Consistency of Psychiatric Ratings

Many studies have dealt with the problem of low consistency of psychiatric ratings with regard to the symptoms and the diagnosis of a patient [3, 4, 16, 17, 22–25]. Besides the general problems of unclear nosological criteria and the complex process of decision-making, there are already considerable difficulties concerning the ratings of a symptom [3, 17, 24]. *Ward* et al. [24] showed in their studies that one third of the disagreement of ratings can be explained by three factors: (1) different interviewing techniques, (2) different weighting of symptoms and (3) different interpretations of the same observation. Similar problems are also stressed in the studies of *Katz* et al. [16] and *Beck* et al. [4]. *Shepherd* et al. [22] showed that the style of the interviewer depends more on experience than on the 'school' he belongs to. They point out the typical mistakes which interfere with the process of decision-making based on the perception of verbal and non-verbal behavior of a patient. They also mentioned the important fact that the interrater reliability on the level of clinical diagnosis is better than the interrater reliability on the level of psychopathological symptoms. Like many other researchers [4, 14, 15]. *Shepherd* et al. [22] stress the importance of an improvement in the common observational language as a result of rater training.

Rating Scales as Instruments for Systematic Observation

Rating scales are specialized complex instruments for systematic observation. Ideally they have to fulfil the requirement that they assess quantitatively operationalized variables. Quantitative assessment of the variables is described in terms of the objectivity, the reliability, and the validity of the instrument. The observer or interviewer should record the relevant observation or data according to the rules of the system and without any distortion by personal characteristics. Such an ideal interview or observation situation, which would be analogous to an experiment, cannot be realized in a clinical setting. Such a restriction of the interview would even make a psychiatric interview impossible. We therefore have to make a compromise between the demands for accuracy and the distorting effects of the situation as well as the personal characteristics of the interviewer [9].

The psychiatric rating situation can be analyzed under the paradigm of social interaction with the goal of reducing data. The interaction between patient and interviewer is characterized by events which have uncertain starting and end points as well as different characteristics. Those events have to be compared with hypothetical dimensions by the interviewer following a set of rules. There are some problems associated with that paradigm [9, 13, 21, 22]: (1) The problem of the explicitness of the rules by which the selection and classification of the data has to be performed, i.e. the quality of the operational definition of the variables. (2) The problem of typical mistakes while interviewing concerning the perceiving, the processing and the recording of the data. Those mistakes concerning the interviewer as a disturbing factor must be limited and controlled.

Concerning the problem of the *perception* of the data, there are processes of attention, saturation and habituation of the interviewer as well as the complexity of the item categories, which might cause mistakes.

Typical errors concerning the *processing* of the data – so-called errors of judgement – are: (1) Errors of central tendency: the interviewer tends to avoid extreme ratings. (2) Errors of leniency or generosity errors: the interviewer's ratings are generally too favorable for the observed subject. (3) Primacy-recency effects: they demonstrate the influence of the 'first impression' of the subject on the interviewer. (4) Halo effects: the interviewer's ratings are distorted by the general impression of the subject or by one or more of the subject's outstanding features. (5) Logical errors: distortions of judgement caused by the interviewer's tendency to rate some items in a similar way because he implicitly assumes a certain correlation between those items. All these effects distort the data and depend on the interview techniques and the training of the rater.

Finally the problem of *recording* the data, which depends on the time interval between the processing and the actual recording. The recording mistakes occur because the interviewer has to deal not only with a complex process of judgement or decision-making, but also with a difficult memory task. Rater training has the objective to reduce the above-mentioned mistakes in order to improve interrater reliability. The less explicit the instructions for observations are, the more the interrater reliability depends on the training of the raters. In that case, the degree of the interrater reliability is more a measure of the effectiveness of the training for a certain rater group than a general measure for the reliability of the instrument.

Because of these problems in the rating process there are two main objectives for rater training [18]. (1) Quantitative discrimination, i. e. after training, the ratings concerning the intensity of a patient's behavior or experience should have a high correlation among raters. (2) Distinction of concepts, i. e. the raters have to learn which behavior or experience of the patient is equivalent to which category in the rating system.

Studies on the Training Effects of the AMDP and Other Rating Scales

There are many studies which stress in a general way the necessity of rater training using films or video recordings [7, 8, 10, 11, 15, 20–22]. However, studies which quantitatively evaluate the effect of training programs are rare [6, 10, 15], and the results of the studies cannot be compared because of the use of different measurements and different statistical procedures.

Von Cranach and Cooper [10] studied the effects of a training program for a standardized interview (PSE). During the training which required 10 ratings per week, some in vivo and some with video recordings, these authors showed that the trainees in comparison to experienced interviewers developped a 'rater bias'. In the beginning of the training the inexperienced interviewers had the tendency to exaggerate pathological symptoms; later in the training the trainees' ratings showed a high correlation with those of the experienced interviewers.

Heimann et al. [15], working with the Hamilton Depression Scale, also studied the training process. The training was extended over 10 months, during which 11 video recordings of depressive patients were shown. *Heimann* et al. [15] also found a significant increase in the correlation between inexperienced and experienced raters at the end of the training.

Training seminars for the AMDP have been investigated by 4 different researchers [2, 6, 7, 11].

Busch et al. [7] used two parameters: the range of the ratings of certain items and a similarity index of the rater profile. During 2 days, 8 video recordings were presented to 21 participants. The first recording was shown a second time at the end of the training period. Concerning the item level two extreme groups were found: one group had a large range and the other group had a small range. The criterium for small range was that no more than 1 rather differed 3 points or no more than 2 raters differed 2 points from the others. During the training the number of items with small ranges increased and the number of items with large ranges decreased. Also the range in some of the remaining items decreased significantly. In the rater profile the similarity increased also; however, a statistically significant result could not be calculated because of methodological reasons.

A decrease in the variance of the raters after retest was also found by *Bobon and von Frenckell* [6] in their study on the French version of the AMDP, trying to use a factor analytical method to measure the distance between the different raters.

Another additional training program to increase the correlation between inexperienced and experienced raters is the use of video recordings which show a standard rating done by experienced interviewers. Those 'video models' are used to teach the techniques of rating and interviewing to inexperienced raters. *Von Cranach and Strauss* [11] have discussed such training programs for the AMDP-System.

With regard to the above-mentioned problems and the results of rater-training programs there are three recommendations for the AMDP-System. These three recommendations are also found in the manual of the AMDP-System, and prove to be realistic and practical training goals for training seminars. (1) Supervision of at least 10 interviews and records by an experienced AMDP interviewer. The interviews should cover the whole range of possible psychiatric symptoms. Therefore, the interviews should be semi-structured and at least 30 min long. Inexperienced as well as experienced interviewers should use the glossary. (2) Films and video recordings should be rated within the group and the differences between the raters should be discussed. (3) Films and video recordings for which standard ratings are available should be used to practice the rating.

References

1 Arbeitsgemeinschaft für Methodik und Dokumentation in der Psychiatrie: Das AMDP-System, 3. Aufl. Springer, Berlin 1979.

2 Baumann, U.; Fähndrich, E.: Recent developments of the AMDP system: AMDP Congress 1980. Pharmakopsychiatr. Neuro-Psychopharmakol. *14:* 74–76 (1981).

3 Beck, A. T.: Reliability of psychiatric diagnoses. 1. A critique of systematic studies. Am. J. Psychiat. *119:* 210–216 (1962).

4 Beck, A. T.; Ward, C. H.; Mendelson, M.; Mock, J. E.; Erbough, J. K.: Reliability of psychiatric diagnoses. 2. A study of consistency of clinical judgements and ratings. Am. J. Psychiat. *119:* 351–357 (1962).

5 Bobon, D. P.: Le système AMDP; 2e éd. (Mardaga, Bruxelles 1981).

6 Bobon, D. P.; v.. Frenckell, R.: Faktorenanalytische Darstellung der Interrater-Reliabilität deutschsprachiger und französischsprachiger AMDP-Rater. AGNP Symposium, Nürnberg, September 1979 (unpublished).

7 Busch, H.; Fähndrich, E.; Freudenthal, K.; Renfordt, E.: Zur Anwendung und Weiterentwicklung des AMDP-Systems. Bericht über ein Symposion und ein Trainingsseminar. Pharmakopsychiatr. Neuro-Psychopharmakol. *7:* 170–175 (1975).

8 Cooper, J. E.; Copeland, J. R. M.; Brown, G. W.; Harris, T.; Gourlay, A. J.: Further studies on interviewer training and inter-rater reliability of the Present State Examination (PSE). Psychol. Med. *7:* 517–523 (1977).

9 Cranach M., v.; Frenz, H. G.: Systematische Beobachtung; in Graumann, Handbuch der Psychologie, Bd. 7, 1. (Hogrefe, Göttingen 1969).

10 Cranach M., v.; Cooper, J. E.: Changes in rating behaviour during the learning of a standardized psychiatric interview. Psychol. Med. *2:* 373–380 (1972).

11 Cranach M., v.; Strauss, A.: Zur Weiterentwicklung des AMDP-Systems. Pharmakopsychiatr. Neuro-Psychopharmakol. *10:* 254–261 (1977).
12 Guy, W.; Ban, T. A: The AMDP system (Springer, New York 1982).
13 Heimann, H.: Psychopathologie; in Kisker, Meyer, Müller, Strömgren, Psychiatrie der Gegenwart, Bd I, 1, 2. Aufl. (Springer, Berlin 1979).
14 Heimann, H.; Angst, J.; Bente, D.; Berner, P.; Helmchen, H.; Hippius, H.: Verbundforschung: Erfahrungen der Arbeitsgemeinschaft für Methodik und Dokumentation in der Psychiatrie (AMP); in Bochnik, Pittrich, Multifaktorielle Probleme in der Psychiatrie (Akad. Verlagsges., Wiesbaden 1976).
15 Heimann, H.; Obermair, W.; Boller, W.; Stoll, K.-D.: Videotape training in psychiatric practice. Prog. Neuro-Psychopharmacol. *1:* 141–145 (1977).
16 Katz, M., Cole, J. O.; Lowery, H. A: Studies of the diagnostic process: the influence of symptom perception, past experience, and ethnic background on diagnostic decisions. Am. J. Psychiat. *125:* 937–947 (1969).
17 Kreitman, N.; Sainsbury, P.; Morrissey, J.; Towers, J.; Scrivener, J.: The reliability of psychiatric assessment: an analysis. J. ment. Sci. *107:* 887–908 (1961).
18 Langer, I.; Schulz v. Thun, F.: Messung komplexer Merkmale in Psychologie und Pädagogik. Ratingverfahren (Reinhardt, Basel 1974).
19 Lopez-Ibor Aliño, J. J.: El sistema AMDP (Grupo para el Progreso de la Psiquiatria, Madrid 1980).
20 Renfordt, E.: Audio-visuelle Methoden in der Psychiatrie. Nervenarzt *45:* 505–509 (1974).
21 Seidenstücker, E.; Seidenstücker, G.: Interviewforschung; in Schraml, Baumann, Klinische Psychologie, II (Huber, Bern 1974).
22 Shepherd, M.; Brooke, E. M.; Cooper, J. E.; Lin, T.: An experimental approach to psychiatric diagnosis. Acta psychiat. scnad. suppl. 201 ad vol. 44 (1968).
23 Temerlin, M. K.: Suggestion effects in psychiatric diagnosis. J. nerv. ment. Dis. *147:* 349–353 (1968).
24 Ward, C. H.; Beck, A. T.; Mendelson, M.; Mock, J. E.; Erbough, J. K.: The psychiatric nomenclature: reasons for diagnostic disagreements. Archs gen. Psychiat. *7:* 198–205 (1962).
25 Zubin, J.: Classification of the behavior disorders. A. Rev. Psychol. *18:* 374–406 (1967).

Prof. H. Heimann, Universitätsnervenklinik, Osianderstrasse 22,
D-7400 Tübingen (FRG)

Mod. Probl. Pharmacopsychiat., vol. 20, pp. 125–142 (Karger, Basel 1983)

Particular Aspects of the Interrater Reliability of the AMDP Psychopathology Scale

E. Renfordt[a], *H. Busch*[a], *M. von Cranach*[b], *W. Gulbinat*[c], *J. Tegeler*[d]

[a] Department of Psychiatry, Free University of Berlin, Berlin, FRG
[b] Department of Psychiatry, University of Munich, Munich, FRG
[c] Division of Mental Health, World Health Organization, Geneva, Switzerland
[d] Department of Psychiatry, University of Düsseldorf, Düsseldorf, FRG

Introduction

The extent of agreement between psychiatric findings obtained by various assessors for the same patient is not at least a question of the used documentation and assessment system. Subsequently interrater reliability tests serve as quality test of the employed instruments of assessment. Some important components influencing overall reliability, however, are left unrecognized if global reliability values are used to demonstrate the rating quality. In this paper we present and discuss some of these components on the basis of the results of a comprehensive interrater reliability study relying on the Association for Methodology and Documentation in Psychiatry (AMP/AMDP) system [8]. Basic aspects of the reliability of the AMP-System have already been published by *Gebhardt and Helmchen* [6], and by *Woggon* et al. [13].

The AMP/AMDP Psychopathological Scale was composed for the documentation of a very broad spectrum of psychopathological symptoms. Since a reliability study can involve examination of only a limited number of patients, we must find out first of all whether the scale of items is covered by the symptoms of this sample of patients. Thus, we must specify the number and type of items for which none of the patients examined showed corresponding symptoms. Of course the relative quantity of the items so defined determines the fundamental value of the test. Regarding reliability, this involves those items for which investigators establish 'absence' with a high degree of agreement for all the patients. This presupposes, however, that we can in general distinguish between high reliability for present symptoms and for absent symptoms. Previous test methods could hardly fulfil this requirement. An effort to solve this problem is attempted in the present paper.

To develop such a strategy is also necessary from a second point of view. The most frequently used statistical concepts of reliability presume that (independently of any statement regarding validity) the absence or presence of a symptom is determined 'correctly' with like probability. Taking into consideration a series of factors involved in the diagnostic process – which we cannot discuss further here – this presupposition must remain basically doubtful. Thus, *Busch and Vogel* [2] have pointed out that particularly in psychopathological examinations false positive judgements are caused by diagnostic factors different from false negative ones. Therefore, the two courses of judgement are subject to different presuppositions of probability. As a consequence of this interpretation it is necessary to differentiate fundamentally between the two reliability statements, i.e. whether the raters agree on the presence or the absence of a symptom.

Thus, if the reliability of an item is investigated in a single patient by a group of assessors one of the following three consequences can result: high reliability for presence, high reliability for absence, or low reliability. Examination of a large number of patients then results in frequency statements for each of these three possibilities. Such a trimodal value utilizes the information content of the ratings more comprehensively, and permits more differentiated conclusions than does a bimodal description (high/low) of the reliability of the item.

Method

Within the context of a multicentre study, 12 video tapes were examined which showed explorations of psychiatric patients; 4 of the patients suffered from schizophrenia, 4 from depressive psychosis and 4 from organic brain disorder. Within the diagnostic groups, half the patients exhibited rather severe symptoms; the symptoms of the other half were less pronounced. Half the tapes were 30 min long, the other half 15 min. They had not been edited or cut. The explorations contained no case history data and were limited to the present symptoms and structured in accordance with AMDP psychopathological and somatic assessment. The tapes were examined in 6 German and Swiss psychiatric centers [Department of Psychiatry, University of Basel, Switzerland; Department of Psychiatry, Free University of Berlin, FRG; Department of Psychiatry, University of Düsseldorf, FRG; Department of Psychiatry, University of Munich, FRG; Max-Planck Institute for Psychiatry, Munich, FRG; Department of Psychiatry, University of Zürich, Switzerland] by a total of 102 assessors. The average psychiatric experience of the assessors was 3.8 years; they had a mean value of 1.6 years experience in using the AMP-System. The tapes were documented with help of a revised version of the 1972 AMP Scales [10] conceived as a draft to the AMDP revision; they contained 115 psychopathological items and 31 somatic ones.

In psychiatry and related disciplines, a number of different coefficients are used for quantifying reliability. Their respective application is determined by theoretical concepts of reliability, the design of the study, the structure of the available data and the aims of investigation. The kappa coefficient is most frequently used in psychiatric reliability problems [5]. Kappa compares the agreement actually reached by 2 or more assessors with the agreement one has to expect by a random model. From the definition of kappa, based on the random model, it results that for low values of kappa no unequivocal interpretation concerning a clear reliability statement is possible. Therefore, in the present investigation we started on a different concept of reliability [7], namely, one which regards the measured value as the sum of the 'true' value and an error component. Here π signifies the probability that the measured value corresponds to the 'true' value. Thus, π becomes a measure of reliability, which is beyond direct calculation insofar as the 'true' value is unknown.

However, if we assume that N assessors ($N > 1$) examine L patients simultaneously and independently of one another and that they agree in M cases, a functional relationship exists between the agreement in judgement a and the measure of reliability π [14].

$$a = \frac{M}{L} = \pi^N + (1-\pi)^N \text{ (dichotomous values),} \tag{1}$$

$$a = \frac{M}{L} = \pi^N + \frac{(1-\pi)^N}{(S-1)^{N-1}} \text{ (polychotomous values with S classes)} \tag{2}$$

With regards to the relationship between a and π it is basically of no account whether reliability is expressed as probability (π) or as the coefficient of agreement (a). The coefficient a_2 used in this study is based upon all possible combinations of pairs of raters and is called the pairwise agreement ratio.

To calculate a_2, we establish first of all – on the basis of the rating result for each item and each patient separately – the number N_+ of assessors who considered a symptom to be present. The number of negative judgement N_- ('symptom absent') is determined in the same way, and the total number of assessors $N_s = N_+ + N_-$. From the values N_s, N_+ and N_- one then calculates the respective maximum possible number of pair combinations according to the general formula of the combinatory analysis:

$$P = \frac{N \cdot (N-1)}{2} . \tag{3}$$

P_+ signifies the total number of possible pair combinations of assessors who agree about the presence of the symptom, and P_- similarly concerning the absence of the symptom. P_s is the total number of possible pair combinations formed from the total number of assessors. The coefficient of agreement a_2 is defined as follows:

$$a_2 = \frac{P_+ + P_-}{P_s} . \tag{4}$$

It is important to note that $P_s = P_+ + P_-$ – and thus $a_2 = 1$ (highest reliability with perfect agreement) – is only possible when either P_+ or P_- assumes the value 0. If this is not the case, $P_s > P_+ + P_-$ and in consequence $a_2 < 1$. Reliability is lowest when $a_2 = 0.5$. This and all the relationships described here presuppose a sufficiently large number of raters, N; in particular, the condition

$$\frac{N-1}{N} \approx 1 \tag{5}$$

must be satisfied. As 102 raters took part in this study, we can regard this condition as being satisfied.

On a high level of reliability the value of a_2 can either support the presence or the absence of the symptom. As mentioned above a decision between these two possibilities, however, is of fundamental concern. A solution can be to form the difference between P_+ and P_- rather than their sum, corresponding to the calculation of a_2. This leads to a new coefficient of agreement r_2, which exhibits a different distribution of values than a_2:

$$r_2 = \frac{P_+ - P_-}{P_s} . \tag{6}$$

The r_2 coefficient varies between +1 und –1. When $r_2 = +1$, there is maximum agreement amongst the investigators in favor of the presence of the symptom; when $r_2 = -1$ the same is the case with respect to the absence of the symptom. Reliability is at its minimum when $r_2 = \pm 0$.

Results

Although some of the results of the study have already been published elsewhere [3, 4], a few of these findings shall be summarized again in the present account.

For the documentation of this assessment five possible alternatives were available to the rater: 'absent', 'no comment', 'mild', 'moderate', 'severe'. The reliability coefficients a_2 were calculated on the basis of this 'original coding', as well as for a 'dichotomous coding' where 'absent' and 'no comment' were set against the judgements 'mild', 'moderate' and 'severe'.

In table I the results are depicted separately for each of the centers. As expected from the smaller range of possible judgements, reliability is distinctly higher with dichotomous coding than with original coding. With dichotomous coding there are no differences worth mentioning between the centers; with original coding, on the other hand, center 2 provides a particularly low value. A controlled follow-up test revealed that the assessors in this center used the assessment 'no comment' more often than 'absent'; in the other centers this assessment was used only in exceptional cases.

A high reliability *within* centers (table I) does not necessarily result in a high reliability *across* centers. When calculating reliability across centers the fact had to be avoided that certain Centers were over-represented or under-represented because of the respective numbers of assessors. Therefore, 6 assessors were selected at random from each Center to form the basis for a joint calculation of reliability. The results were controlled on further random samples. The findings are given in table II. Whilst no difference was observed with dichotomous coding, with original coding reliability within Centers was slightly higher than reliability across Centers. By means of factor analysis particular components of agreement in judgement were found between two Centers which work in close mutual cooperation [3, 4].

Essential findings for the somatic AMDP are summarized in ta-

Table I. Mean a_2 values of each Center for original and dichotomous coding; AMDP Psychopathology Scale (all raters)

	Reliability (a_2) original coding	Reliability (a_2) dichotomous coding
Center 1	0.80	0.87
Center 2	0.74	0.86
Center 3	0.81	0.86
Center 4	0.80	0.86
Center 5	0.78	0.85
Center 6	0.78	0.88
Mean	0.79	0.86

Table II. Mean a_2 values within and across Centers for original and dichotomous coding; AMDP Psychopathology Scale (6 raters from each Center)

	Reliability (a_2) within centers	Reliability (a_2) across centers
Original coding	0.79	0.76
Dichotomous coding	0.86	0.86

Table III. Mean a_2 values within and across Centers for original and dichotomous coding; AMDP Scale for somatic symptoms

	Reliability (a_2) within centers	Reliability (a_2) across centers
Original coding	0.59	0.53
Dichotomous coding	0.95	0.95

ble III. It can be seen that the somatic reliability values are strikingly low for tests both within and across centers when original coding data are evaluated, being dinstinctly lower than the corresponding values from psychopathological findings. On the other hand, dichotomous evaluation produces reliability values even higher than those achieved with psychopathological findings. This discrepancy between psychopathological and somatic findings is explained by the more frequent use of the assessment category 'no comment' as opposed to 'absent' in the case of somatic

Table IV. Mean a_2 value and standard deviations for each patient; AMDP Psychopathology Scale

Diagnosis	Patient No.	a_2	s
Schizophrenia	1	0.77	0.19
	2	0.84	0.17
	3	0.82	0.17
	4	0.83	0.18
	$\bar{x}$	0.82	
Depressive psychosis	5	0.85	0.17
	6	0.88	0.17
	7	0.87	0.17
	8	0.90	0.17
	$\bar{x}$	0.88	
Organic brain disorder	9	0.91	0.15
	10	0.87	0.18
	11	0.85	0.18
	12	0.87	0.17
	$\bar{x}$	0.88	
Total	$\bar{x}$	0.86	

items. Thus, the assessors did not agree in distinguishing between these two assessment categories. The information from the TV tapes, which formed the basis of assessment, was clearly inappropriate for bringing out this distinction as regards somatic findings.

We will first consider results on the level of the individual patient. The problem of separate reliability tests for present and absent symptoms will be discussed in this context. These evaluations are limited to psychopathological AMDP findings and to the dichotomous coding.

Table IV gives a survey of the reliability results for each individual patient. With the exception of patient 1 (schizophrenia) all values are of sufficiently high reliability with little variation. There are no differences worth mentioning between the three diagnostic groups.

In order to check whether the high a_2 reliability values depend on agreement concerning present or absent symptoms, figure 1 gives the frequency distribution of r_2 values, averaged over all 12 patients examined for consecutively defined reliability classes. It is evident that the frequency of r_2 values in the left area of distribution $(-1.0 \le r_2 < -0.8)$

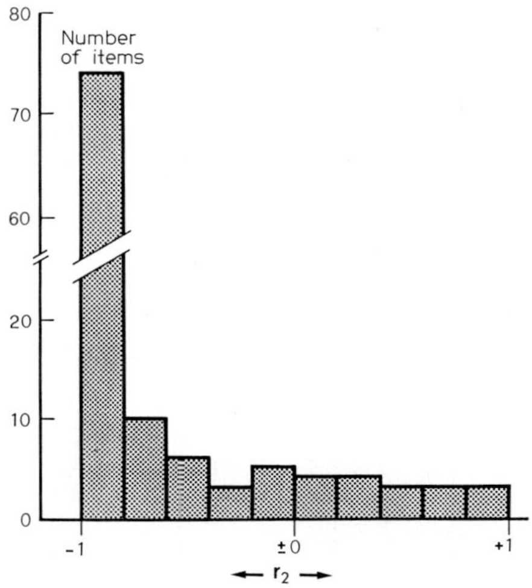

Fig. 1. Frequency distribution of all items of the AMDP Psychopathology Scale in reference to their r_2-values (mean value per patient).

Table V. Mean r_2 value and standard deviations for each patient; AMDP Psychopathology Scale

Diagnosis	Patient No.	r_2	s
Schizophrenia	1	– 0.48	0.56
	2	– 0.65	0.51
	3	– 0.64	0.49
	4	– 0.63	0.53
	$\bar{x}$	– 0.60	
Depressive psychosis	5	– 0.60	0.59
	6	– 0.71	0.51
	7	– 0.71	0.49
	8	– 0.75	0.48
	$\bar{x}$	– 0.69	
Organic brain disorder	9	– 0.76	0.50
	10	– 0.65	0.57
	11	– 0.62	0.56
	12	– 0.70	0.51
	$\bar{x}$	– 0.68	
Total	$\bar{x}$	– 0.66	

which characterizes the class with the highest reliability values for absence, is by far the highest: 74 (about 64%) of the 115 items of the scale belong to this category alone. The remaining items are distributed over the other classes without any clear distinction. It follows that the high global reliability values (a_2) depend almost exclusively on a high rate of agreement as regards the absence of symptoms. Neither in the area of low reliability (around $r_2 = \pm 0$) nor in the area of high reliability for present symptoms (towards $r_2 = +1$) one finds a frequency increase which would serve to characterize a corresponding category of items.

The r_2 values for each patient assembled in table V also correspond to this result. Except for patient 1, they all indicate a sufficiently high reliability for absent symptoms ($r_2 < -0.5$).

As a consequence of this result we made a controlled search for items of specially low reliability and for those with high reliability for presence. Table VI examines for each of the 115 items of the scale the frequency with which they fall in the three possible classes of reliability for all 12 patients. These three reliability classes were defined as follows: high reliability for presence ($0.5 \leq r_2 \leq +1$), high reliability for absence ($-0.5 \geq r_2 \geq -1$), low reliability ($-0.5 < r_2 < +0.5$). Note that in conformity with conservative strategy, the area of low reliability is designed twice as large as the two areas of high reliability.

Thus, each item acquires a 3-dimensional value, giving differential characterization of its reliability. A count of table VI reveals that not less than 50 items on the scale fall, for at least 1 patient, within the area of high reliability for presence (table VII). On the other hand, the corresponding values for low reliability is 78 items; for high reliability for absence it is 114 items (the item 'concentration disorders' alone is missing here). At the level of the individual patient the values are assembled correspondingly in table VIII. Differences between patients (again except for patient 1) and diagnostic groups are small. On the average, for each patient 8 items are established with high reliability as present, 20 as with low reliability and 87 as absent with high reliability.

The complex structure of all these data means that we have to look for ways of representing and summarizing clearly the essential elements of the overall result of the study. Topological configuration analysis is particularly appropriate here.

As we see from table VI each item on the psychopathological AMDP Scale is defined by three frequency components: the number of patients for whom absence was recorded with sufficient reliability, the frequency

Table VI. Distribution into three reliability classes of each item of the AMDP Psychopathology Scale for 12 patients examined

	High reliability for absence	Low reliability	High reliability for presence
I. Disorders of consciousness			
1 Clouded consciousness	12	0	0
2 Delirious	11	0	1
3 Twilight state	12	0	0
4 Confusional state	11	1	0
II. Disturbances of orientation			
5 Time	9	1	2
6 Place	11	0	1
7 Situation	11	0	1
8 Self	12	0	0
9 Double orientation	12	0	0
III. Disorders of attention and memory			
10 Apperception	8	3	1
11 Concentration	0	6	6
12 Acquisition	8	1	3
13 Retention	6	3	3
14 Confabulation	10	0	2
15 Paramnesias	12	0	0
IV. Formal disturbances of thinking			
16 Inhibition	8	4	0
17 Blocking	12	0	0
18 Retardation	5	4	3
19 Restriction	2	9	1
20 Circumstantial	10	1	1
21 Perseveration	10	2	0
22 Acceleration/flight of ideas	8	2	2
23 Paralogia (tangential talk)	8	4	0
24 Incoherence	8	4	0
25 Thought stopping	9	3	0
26 Pressured	9	3	0
V. Fears, overvalued ideas, obsessions			
27 Hypochondriasis (not delusional)	12	0	0
28 Overvalued ideas	12	0	0
29 Obsessive symptoms	12	0	0
30 Phobias	12	0	0
31 Impulsive actions	12	0	0

Table VI. (contd.)

	high reliability for absence	low reliability	high reliability for presence
VI. Delusions			
32 Delusional mood	8	2	2
33 Delusional perception	8	3	1
34 Delusional irruption	7	2	3
35 Systematized delusion	8	2	2
36 Delusional dynamic	7	2	3
37 Delusions of reference	8	2	2
38 Phantastic delusion	11	1	0
39 Delusions of grandeur	10	1	1
40 Delusions of persecution	8	3	1
41 Delusions of love	12	0	0
42 Delusions of guilt	11	0	1
43 Delusions of impoverishment	12	0	0
44 Hypochondriacal delusions	12	0	0
VII. Disorders of perception			
45 Illusions	11	1	0
46 Verbal hallucinations	9	2	1
47 Other auditory hallucinations	11	1	0
48 Visual hallucinations	8	2	2
49 Bodily hallucinations	9	1	2
50 Olfactory/gustatory hallucinations	11	0	1
51 Pseudohallucinations	12	0	0
VIII. Disorders of ego			
52 Depersonalization	8	3	1
53 Derealization	9	3	0
54 Autism	10	2	0
55 Thought broadcasting	11	1	0
56 Thought withdrawal	10	2	0
57 Thought insertion	8	2	2
58 Other symptoms of being influenced	9	2	1
59 Apersonalization/transitivism	12	0	0
IX. Disorders of affect			
60 Perplexity	2	10	0
61 Indifferent	9	3	0
62 Feeling of loss of feeling	8	4	0
63 Disturbances of vital feelings	6	4	2

Table VI. (contd.)

	high reliability for absence	low reliability	high reliability for presence
IX. Disorders of affect (contd.)			
64 Depression	4	2	6
65 Hopelessness	7	3	2
66 Anxiety	4	7	1
67 Euphoria	8	4	0
68 Irritability	10	2	0
69 Suspiciousness	9	3	0
70 Tension	6	5	1
71 Inner restlessness	1	8	3
72 Complaintiveness	9	3	0
73 Silly; fatuous	12	0	0
74 Ecstasy	12	0	0
75 Feelings of inadequacy	5	3	4
76 Exaggerated self-confidence	9	1	2
77 Feelings of guilt	8	3	1
78 Feelings of impoverishment	11	1	0
79 Ambivalence	9	3	0
80 Inadequate affect	7	5	0
81 Emotional lability	9	3	0
82 Emotional incontinence	10	1	1
83 Emotional rigidity	3	9	0
84 Tenacity of affects	12	0	0
X. Disturbances of drive and psychomotility			
85 Lack of drive	4	4	4
86 Inhibition of drive	7	5	0
87 Indecisive	8	4	0
88 Stupor	12	0	0
89 Mutism	12	0	0
90 Increased drive	8	3	1
91 Motor restlessness	5	5	2
92 Parakinesis	11	1	0
93 Negativism	12	0	0
94 Mannerism	12	0	0
95 Logorrhea	9	2	1
96 Perseveration (motor)	12	0	0
XI. Circadian disturbances			
97 Worse in am	12	0	0
98 Worse in pm	10	0	0
99 Better in pm	12	0	0
100 Alternating	12	0	0

Table VI. (contd.)

	high reliability for absence	low reliability	high reliability for presence
XII. Other disturbances			
101 Reduced social contact	6	5	1
102 Excessive social contact	11	1	0
103 Feeling of illness	5	3	4
104 Lack of feeling of illness	7	4	1
105 Lack of insight of illness	6	4	2
106 Refusal of treatment	11	1	0
107 Suicidal tendencies	9	2	1
108 Suicidal actions	10	1	1
109 Self-mutilation tendencies	12	0	0
110 Aggressiveness	10	2	0
111 Exaggerated sexual drive	12	0	0
112 Reduced sexual drive	10	1	1
113 Difficulty in employment	3	9	0
114 Refusal of eating	12	0	0
115 Lack of self-care	12	0	0

Table VII. Number of items of the AMDP Psychopathology Scale in three reliability classes for at least 1 patient examined

	Number of items	Percent of 115 items
High reliability for absence	114	99
Low reliability	78	68
High reliability for presence	50	43

of its reliable presence, and finally the frequency of its unreliable occurrence. Since the sum of these three frequencies amounts in each case to 12 (12 patients being examined), the total number of possible frequency combinations for a single item is limited, and – as is shown by systematic permutation – comes to 91. We can now construct a triangle of 91 cells whose corners represent the three classes of reliability in question (fig. 2). Each item is now coordinated with its appropriate cell in accordance with the frequencies recorded for it in respect to the three defined classes of reliability. The extent to which the cells are filled represents therefore the number of items which occur with the frequency pattern defined by

Table VIII. Frequency distribution of the 115 items into three reliability classes for each of the patients examined

Diagnosis	Patient No.	High reliability for absence	Low reliability	High reliability for presence
Schizophrenia	1	68	36	11
	2	88	18	9
	3	84	23	8
	4	87	21	7
	$\bar{x}$	82	25	9
Depressive psychosis	5	87	17	11
	6	90	17	8
	7	92	17	6
	8	94	17	4
	$\bar{x}$	91	17	7
Organic brain disorder	9	96	12	7
	10	86	19	10
	11	82	25	8
	12	92	16	7
	$\bar{x}$	89	18	8
Total	$\bar{x}$	87	20	8

these cells. A similar mode of representation is in use in geology for petrological classification in terms of three mineral components [11].

Which attributes in particular are exhibited by the triangle represented in figure 2? The corner cells are occupied when one of the three reliability classes occurs with maximum frequency, i.e. when the item falls within the class in question for all 12 patients, the other two classes being empty. The bordering cells of the triangle contain only two of the reliability classes; the third class is not represented. For all internal cells of the triangle the three reliability classes are represented in the result. The greater the frequency with which an item falls within the area of non-reliability, the further its upward movement in the pyramid, and vice versa. The horizontal row of cells gives the frequency relationship between high reliability for presence (right) and for absence (left).

When all 115 items have been entered in the triangle, a striking accumulation of frequency is discovered in the lower left area, thus in the re-

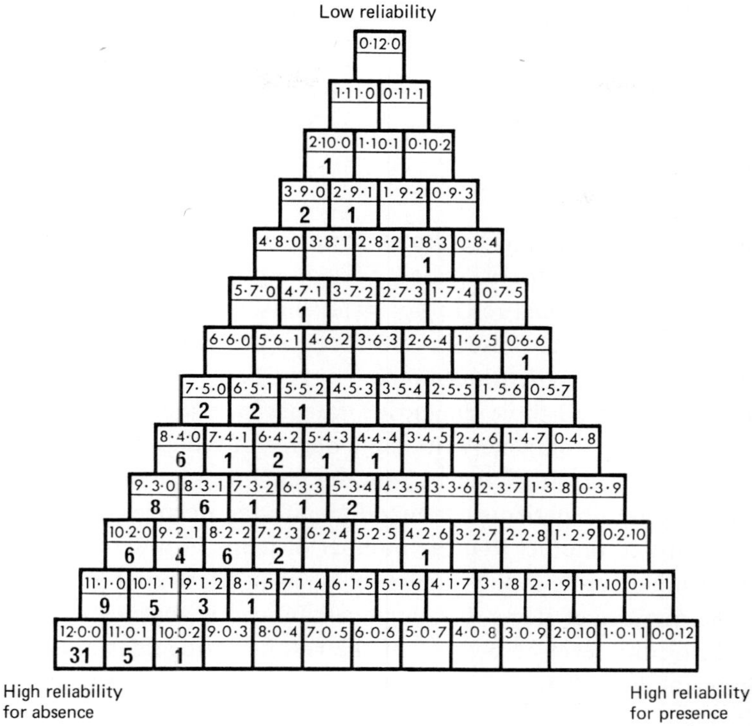

Fig. 2. Distribution of items in a three-dimensional field; entries in the cells signify item frequencies; in the cell index, the first number signifies the frequency of reliable judgements of absence, the middle number the frequency of unreliable values and the last number the frequency of reliable judgements of presence of symptoms.

gion of high reliability for absence. As regards the zones of transition to the other two reliability classes, a considerable occupation of cells is apparent in the direction of low reliability (left marginal cells), whilst high reliability for presence occurs for the most part only together with the other two reliability classes (interior cells). In the upper area of the triangle we find an accumulation of a few items which were found with particular frequency as not very reliable. Amongst these we find: 'perplexity', 'restricted thinking'. 'affective rigidity', 'decreased activities', 'inner restlessness', 'anxiety'. An isolated item on the right hand margin of the triangle ('concentration disorders') appears 6 times with low reliability and 6 times with high reliability for presence; in contrast to all other items of the scale it never occurred as highly reliable for absence. Further details can also be deduced from this trigram, in conjunction with table VI.

Discussion

What conclusions can be drawn from the results for evaluating the psychopathological AMDP Scale? This question can be answered beyond the scope of global reliability statements as a result of the distinction made between the presence and absence of items of high reliability for each individual patient examined.

Patients from all three diagnostic categories examined could be represented with approximately the same degree of reliability. Even within the diagnostic groups differences between patients were slight. Only 1 of the 4 schizophrenic patients examined manifested decreased overall reliability, owing to the fact that the number of items of low reliability was high in comparison with the number of items of high reliability for presence; the number of items with high reliability for absence for this patient was on the level of the rest of the results. Altogether, the psychopathological AMDP Scale satisfies the aim of working independently of any particular given syndrome.

According to high reliability assessment by the investigators, 31 of the 115 items of the scale were found with none of the 12 patients examined. Thus, 27 % of the scale has not been covered by corresponding symptoms on the TV tapes within the context of this study. With only 12 patients examined this result must be regarded as satisfactory especially in the context of a controlled selection of patients with a broad scattering of their psychopathological symptoms. It is worth noting that the 31 items mentioned above were judged to be absent by the assessors on a high level of agreement. Thus, their reliability for absence can be regarded as established, whereas their reliability for presence could not be tested here.

Considering the entire sample of patients the frequency of sufficiently reliable judgements of absence proved to be extremely high in comparison with judgements of presence. This result was to be expected, for the symptoms of each individual patient corresponded to only a fraction of the scale, and the remainder of the items (87 items on average – table V) were not positively marked. In the case of a scale which is independent of any particular given syndrome, such as the AMDP-System, this component of items must be particularly large from the outset. But precisely in this connection it becomes particularly clear how questionable it is to have the high reliability of these (absent) items influence a global reliability judgement of the scale. These items should be regarded as the quasi-negative screen against which we project a positive picture of the patient's symptoms. Therefore, it is not an insignificant factor that these items were established with high reliability (as absent). This reliability states quite a different situation from that described by a high reliability for presence of a symptom.

On average, 20 items per patient were found with low reliability and 8 items with high reliability for presence (table VIII). This ratio, which may appear unfavorable at first sight, presumably has its cause in a series of factors which work jointly to the same end, and which relativize an assessment of the scale on the basis of results:

(1) This investigation was realized as a multicenter study in 6 different centers in 2 countries. Because of this widely scattered and heterogeneous sample of assessors, expectations were limited from the start about achieving a particularly high reliability.

(2) The demarcation between the three reliability classes in respect of r_2 values was made schematically, but using conservative strategy. A modification of these limits would result in modification of the frequency distribution in the question here.

(3) TV assessments offer the advantage that a large number of investigators can judge identical psychopathological phenomena [9]. The question is, however, to what extent TV assessments, compared with original exploration, can negatively influence a reliability result. As the TV assessor has no chance to investigate by extensive exploration the symptoms which appear to him doubtful concerning presence or absence, the frequency of low reliability findings could be increased for many raters. Particularly symptoms which stand (as regards intensity) on the threshold of being definitely perceptible should show this effect. However, this disagrees with the fact that in the present study neither the patients with the more severe or the slighter symptoms nor the 15- or 30-min explorations led to any differences in reliability worth mentioning.

The present study was intended to provide an empirical basis for the revision of the psychopathological AMDP Scale. The results of the study have meanwhile received attention in the revised 3rd edition of the AMDP-System [1]. The items which continuously showed low reliability (fig. 2) were redefined or deleted. In this way the overall reliability of the scale should have been further improved.

Acknowledgements

The authors wish to thank Prof. *J. Angst* (Zürich), Prof. *H. Helmchen* (Berlin) and Prof. *N. Sartorius* (Geneva) for the first idea and the conceptual design of the study. We are also indept to all raters participating in the study and to *H. Kluge* for his technical assistance.

References

1 Arbeitsgemeinschaft für Methodik und Dokumentation in der Psychiatrie: Das AMDP-System: 3. Aufl. (Springer, Berlin 1979).

2 Busch, H.; Vogel, H.-P., Differences in the documentation of psychopathological assessment: free text versus rating scale (AMP-form 3). Meth. Inform. Med. *16:* 131–137 (1977).

3 Busch, H.; Cranach, M. v.; Gulbinat, W.; Renfordt, E.; Tegeler, J., Reliability of the AMDP-System. Acta psychiat. scand. *62:* 382–392 (1980).

4 Busch, H.; Cranach, M.; Gulbinat, W.; Renfordt, E.; Tegeler, J., Methodological and practical aspects of a multicenter approach on the reliability of psychopathological assessment; in Sartorius, Helmchen, Multicenter trials (Karger, Basel 1981).

5 Cohen, J., A coefficient of agreement for nominal scales. Educ. psychol. Measur. *20:* 37–46 (1960).

6 Gebhardt, R.; Helmchen, H., Zur Zuverlässigkeit psychopathologischer Symptomerfassung. Die Übereinstimmung mehrerer Beurteiler im AMP-System. Schweiz. Arch. Neurol. Neurochir. Psychiat. *112:* 459–469 (1973).

7 Guilford, J. P.; Psychometric methods; 2nd ed. (McGraw Hill, New York 1954).

8 Helmchen, H.; The AMP system as a method in clinical pharmacopsychiatry; in Hippius, Assessment of pharmacodynamic effects in human pharmacology, pp. 87–134 (Schattauer, Stuttgart 1975).

9 Helmchen, H.; Renfordt, E., The contribution of audio-visual techniques to advance in psychopathology. Compreh. Psychiat. *22:* 21–30 (1981).

10 Scharfetter, C. (ed.), Das AMP-System. Manual zur Dokumentation psychiatrischer Befunde; 2nd ed. (Springer, Berlin 1972).

11 Streckeisen, A., Classification and nomenclature of Igneous Rocks. N. JB. Mineral. Abh. *107:* 144–240 (1967).

12 Wing, J. K.; Cooper, J. E.; Sartorius, N., The measurement and classification of psychiatric symptoms (Cambridge University Press, Cambridge 1974).

13 Woggon, B.; Baumann, U.; Angst, J., Interrater-Reliabilität von AMP-Symptomen. Arch. Psychiat. Nerv. Krankh. *225:* 73–85 (1978).

14 World Health Organization, Schizophrenia. An international follow-up study (Wiley & Sons, Chichester 1979).

E. Renfordt, MD, Dept. of Psychiatry, Free University of Berlin, Eschenallee 3, D-1000 Berlin 19 (FRG)

Mod. Probl. Pharmacopsychiat., vol. 20, pp. 143–160 (Karger, Basel 1983)

Interrater Reliability of AMDP and AMP Symptoms

S. Kuny, N. von Luckner, R. Baenninger, P. Baur, G. Eichenberger, B. Woggon

Research Department, Psychiatric University Hospital Zürich, Zürich, Switzerland

Introduction

The Association for Methodology and Documentation in Psychiatry (AMP) system has been widely used for a standardized documentation of psychopathological symptoms [*Angst* et al., 1969; *Scharfetter,* 1972]. In 1979 a new version was published under a new set of initials: AMDP. The new version is the result of many years of intensive research. A detailed description of the differences between the two versions is outlined by *Fähndrich* et al. [this volume]. An important criterion for the quality of a rating scale is the interrater reliability. Therefore, we compared the interrater reliability of the AMP and AMDP-Systems.

Methodology

Description of the Raters

The study was carried out by three residents and a psychologist working at the Research Department of the Psychiatric University Hospital Zürich. Before the beginning of the study they had already practised the use of the AMP-System. After each training interview the differences between the two versions were thoroughly discussed.

Selection of Patients

The sample includes mainly schizophrenic and depressed patients (table I), resulting in a close similarity to patients who are treated in our psychopharmacological trials. Based on the number of four raters it was

Table I. Diagnoses (ICD-9)

ICD No.	Diagnosis	n total	Schizophrenic syndrome	Depressive syndrome
295.0	Schizophrenic psychosis, simple type	1		1
295.1	Schizophrenic psychosis, hebephrenic type	1	1	
295.3	Schizophrenic psychosis, paranoid type	16	15	1
295.4	Acute schizophrenic episode	2	2	
295.7	Schizophrenic psychosis, schizoaffective type	7	3	4
296.1	Manic-depressive psychosis, depressed type	11	1	10
296.2	Manic-depressive psychosis, circular type but currently manic	1		1
296.3	Manic-depressive psychosis, circular type but currently depressed	5		5
298.1	Other nonorganic psychosis, excitation type	1	1	
300.4	Neurotic depression	1		1
301.5	Hysterical personality disorder	1	1	
309.1	Prolonged depressive reaction	1		1
		48	24	24

possible to work with six pairs of raters who interviewed 48 patients in a randomized order.

Performance of the Interviews

Patients were selected by doctors who did not participate in the interviews. Each patient was interviewed by one investigator [interviewer] in the presence of another investigator [rater]. The interview referred to the symptomatology of the patient during the last 24 h. After the exploration interviewer and rater documented the symptomatology separately using two sheets of the AMP and AMDP-System for psychopathological symptoms and somatic signs. In addition some statements concerning the interview and the case history of the patient were documented. The duration of the interviews was on average 35 min (s = 9.1, range 20–60 min).

Table II. Number of symptoms with different interrater reliability in AMDP and AMP-Systems

Interrater reliability category	Kappa significant $p \leq 0.1$	Agreement percentage AP	AMDP number	%*	%**	AMP number	%*	%**
Good								
A	≥ 0.6 s.	≥ 80%	43	31.6	53.1	41	22.7	49.4
Moderate								
B1	0.4–0.59 s.	≥ 80%	13 } 25	18.4	30.9	13 } 25	13.8	30.1
B2		70 ≤ AP < 80%	12			12		
Poor								
C	≤ 0.4 s./n. s.	< 80%	13	9.6	16.0	17	9.4	20.5
Cannot be judged								
D1	≥ 0.4 n. s.	≥ 80%	4					
D2	< 0.4 s./n. s.	≥ 80%	20 } 55	40.4		98	54.1	
D3	cannot be judged because marginal total zero		32					
			136	100	100	181	100	100

%* Refers to all items.
%** Refers to rateable items only.

Data Analysis

The choice of statistical methods for data analysis of studies on interrater reliability is determined by the number of raters, number of patients, number and scale niveau of the items [*Langer and Schulz von Thun,* 1974; *Tinsley and Weiss,* 1975]. Dichotomized AMP items are nominal data. Therefore, we used the kappa coefficient [*Cohen,* 1960, 1972; *significance test: Everitt,* 1968; *Fleiss* et al., 1969]. Kappa shows the relation of real agreements between raters to the number of agreements which could be expected by chance. Kappa varies between +1 (total agreement) and –1 (no agreement at all). If the agreement between raters cannot be differentiated from the agreement expected by chance kappa is 0. Kappa was calculated using a table with four fields: symptom present (+) versus symptom not present (–). In addition the percentage of agree-

Table III. Interrater reliability of new AMDP[1] items

Interrater reliability good category A	20	rumination
	104	early waking
	127	backache
Interrater reliability cannot be judged category D_1, D_2, D_3	21	pressured thinking
	14	paramnesias
	86	histrionics
	90	worse in the evening
	114	gastric discomfort
	128	heaviness in the legs
	131	conversion symptoms

[1] In all tables based on the translation of *Guy and Ban* [1982]

ment (fields ++ and −−, related to N] was calculated. A more detailed description is given in *Woggon* et al. [1978]. Based on kappa, its significance and the percentage of agreement the quality of the interrater reliability was classified using four categories (table II).

Description of the Patients

The sample includes 26 female and 22 patients with a mean age of $\bar{x} = 42.4$ ($s = 16.4$) years (range 19–75 years). The duration of illness since the first manifestation was on average $\bar{x} = 8.5$ years ($s = 8.9$, max. = 41); 6 patients showed a first manifestation of their illness. In 29 patients the symptomatology had developed during less than a month before hospitalization. The other 19 patients had already symptoms since more than 6 months. The duration of their stay in hospital until the day of the interview was on average $\bar{x} = 55.4$ days ($s = 175.7$, range 1–1,095). On the day of the interview 41 patients were already treated with psychotropic drugs: antipsychotic drugs ($n = 29$), antiparkinsonian drugs ($n = 9$), antidepressants ($n = 16$) or other psychopharmacological drugs ($n = 11$): 34 patients showed a distinct to extreme severeness of their illness and 14 only a slight to moderate severity. Table I shows the diagnoses of the patients and whether a schizophrenic or depressive syndrome was present on the day of the interview.

Table IV. Interrater reliability (IRR) of AMDP and AMP[1] items with different content: AMDP = AMP

Category	AMDP	Category	AMP
A	54 depersonalization	A	54 disturbance of ego-identity
A	45 delusions of grandeur	A	42 delusions of grandeur
A	80 lack of drive	A	87 lack of initiative and spontaneity
			89 stuporous, IRR not judgeable
A	95 suicidal tendencies	A	109 suicidal tendencies
			110 suicidal acts, IRR not judgeable
A	109 decreased libido[2]	A	115 decreased sexual drive
B1	9 disturbances of apperception	B1	10 disorders of apperception
B1	51 bodily hallucinations	B1	51 body hallucinations
B1	59 perplexity	B1	62 perplexed
B2	18 restricted thinking	B2	19 restricted

[1] In all tables based on the translation of *Helmchen* [1975].
[2] Kappa significantly different ($p \leq 0.05$).

Table V. Quality of interrater reliability of AMDP and AMP items with different content: AMDP > AMP

Category	AMDP	Category	AMP
A	135 acute dyskinesia	D1	173 paroxysmal dyskinesia
		D2	174 persistent hyperkinesia
A	134 tremor[1]	B2	170 fine tremor
		D2	171 medium or gross tremor
B1	11 disturbance of memorization	D2	12 disorders of attention and immediate memory
B1	25 incoherence	D2	24 incoherent/confused
C	10 disturbances of concentration	D2	11 disorders of concentration
C	24 blocking	D2	17 blocking
		C	25 thought-stopping

[1] Kappa significantly different ($p \leq 0.05$).

Table VI. Quality of interrater reliability of AMDP and AMP items with different content: AMDP < AMP

Category	AMDP	Category	AMP
B1	55 thought broadcasting	A	57 broadcasting of thoughts
B1	71 feelings of inadequacy	A	77 feeling of insufficiency, inadequacy
C	12 disturbances of retention	A	13 disorders of memory
D1	94 aggressiveness	A	112 aggressive tendencies
D2	22 flight of ideas	B1	22 accelerated/flight of ideas

Table VII. Interrater reliability of AMDP and AMP items with different content. Interrater reliability in AMDP and AMP-Systems not judgeable (category D1, D2, D3)

AMDP	AMP
1 lowered vigilance	1 clouded consciousness
	4 other disorders of consciousness
2 clouded consciousness	2 delirious
3 narrowed consciousness	3 twilight state
4 expanded consciousness	76 ecstatic
7 disturbances of orientation regarding the situation	7 disorders of orientation regarding the situation
44 hypochondriacal delusions	40 hypochondriacal delusions
53 derealization	55 other experiences of alienation/derealization
84 parakinesia	93 parakinesis/stereotypy
190 lack of self-care	118 patient has to be fed
	119 patient has to be taken care of regarding personal hygiene
	120 incontinent of urine and feces

Table VIII. Interrater reliability of AMDP and AMP items with different names

Category	AMDP	Category	AMP
AMDP = AMP			
A	63 depressed mood	A	66 depressed/sad
A	64 hopelessness	A	67 hopeless/desperate
A	66 euphoria	A	69 elated/euphoric
C	61 blunted affect	C	63 blunted affect
AMDP > AMP			
A	76 parathymia	B1	82 inadequate affect

Table IX. Interrater reliability of AMDP and AMP item with different names. Interrater reliability in AMDP and AMP-Systems not judgeable (category D1, D2, D3)

AMDP	AMP
26 neologisms	96 disorganized speech/neologism
85 mannerisms	95 mannerisms
92 social withdrawal	103 reduced contact
93 excessive social contact	104 increased contact
132 hypertonia	168 increased muscle tone

Results

Mainly due to the small number (n = 48) and diagnostic selection of patients the percentage of items whose interrater reliability could not be calculated was relatively high: 40.4% (AMDP) and 54.1% (AMP). We were especially interested in the interrater reliability of items which are different in both versions. Firstly there are 10 new items in the AMDP-System. The interrater reliability could only be judged for three of them (table III), showing a good quality. Secondly, 29 items of the AMP-System have been changed in the AMDP-System regarding their content and partially their name. They were compared with the matching symptoms of the AMP-System (table IV–VII). Nine items showed in both versions the same interrater reliability, six items a better one in the AMDP-System and five a better one in the AMP-System. For nine items kappa could not be calculated.

Thirdly, for 10 items only the name has been changed. Four show in both versions the same interrater reliability, one a better one in the AMDP-System and for five the interrater reliability could not be calculated (tables VIII, IX).

Tables X and XI list together all items of the AMP-System and AMDP-System with their kappa, significancy and percentage of agreement.

Table X. AMP symptoms

Item No.	Item	Kappa	Significant	Agreement	Category
Disorders of consciousness					
1	Clouded consciousness			96	D_3
2	Delirious				D_3
3	Twilight state			98	D_3
4	Other				D_3
Disorders of orientation					
5	In time	0.90	**	98	A
6	In place			98	D_3
7	Regarding the situation				D_3
8	In person				D_3
9	Other				D_3
Disorders of attention and memory					
10	Disorders of apperception (grasp)	0.54	*	94	B^1
11	Disorders of concentration	0.33	*	83	D_2
12	Disorders of attention and immediate memory	0.39		90	D_2
13	Disorders of memory	0.62	**	81	A
14	Confabulations				D_3
15	Other			98	D_3
Formal disturbances of thinking					
16	Inhibited	0.48	**	77	B_2
17	Blocked	0.33		88	D_2
18	Retarded	0.62	**	81	A
19	Restricted	0.54	**	77	B_2
20	Circumstantial	0.10		73	C
21	Perseverating	–0.04		92	D_2
22	Accelerated/flight of ideas	0.49	**	90	B_1
23	Paralogia (tangential talk)	0.50	**	79	B_2
24	Incoherent/confused	0.12		83	D_2
25	Thought stopping	0.37	**	71	C
26	Other	0.12		83	D_2
Overvalued ideas, compulsions, phobias					
27	Hypochondriasis (not delusional)			98	D_3
28	Overvalued ideas			98	D_3
29	Obsessive thoughts	0.37		94	D_2
30	Compulsive impulses	–0.02		96	D_2
31	Compulsive actions			98	D_3
32	Phobias				D_3
33	Other disturbances				D_3

Table X. AMP symptoms (contd.)

Item No.	Item	Kappa	Significant	Agreement	Category
Delusion					
34	Delusional mood	0.75	**	88	A
35	Delusional perceptions	–0.03		73	D_2
36	Delusional ideation/ delusional thoughts	0.52	**	77	B_2
37	Delusional dynamics	0.50	**	79	B_2
38	Systematized delusions	0.58	**	85	B_2
39	Delusions of guilt	0.26		90	D_2
40	Hypochondriacal delusions				D_3
41	Delusions of poverty			98	D_3
42	Delusions of grandeur	0.81	**	96	A
43	Delusions of reference	0.56	**	81	B_1
44	Delusions of persecution	0.65	**	83	A
45	Delusions of jealousy				D_3
46	Other delusions			92	D_3
Disorders of perception					
47	Illusions			96	D_3
48	Hallucinations of voices	0.89	**	96	A
49	Other auditory hallucinations	1.00	**	100	A
50	Visual hallucinations	0.65	**	96	A
51	Body hallucinations	0.45	**	85	B_1
52	Olfactory and gustatory hallucinations	1.oo	*	100	A
53	Other disorders				D_3
Disorders of ego and personality					
54	Disturbance of ego-identity	0.77	**	94	A
55	Other experiences of alienation/derealization	0.23		90	D_2
56	Autism	0.14		69	C
57	Broadcasting of thoughts	0.60	**	85	A
58	Thought withdrawal	–0.03		90	D_2
59	Thought insertion	0.56	**	83	B_1
60	Other experiences of being influenced by an alien force	0.24		75	C
61	Other			98	D_3

Table X. AMP symptoms (contd.)

Item No.	Item	Kappa	Significant	Agreement	Category
Mood disorders; emotional disturbances					
62	Perplexed	0.41	**	81	B_1
63	Blunted affect	0.13		58	C
64	Feeling of affective coldness	0.48	**	77	B_2
65	Disturbance of vital feelings	0.49	**	75	B_2
66	Depressed/sad	0.95	**	98	A
67	Hopeless/desperate	0.62	**	81	A
68	Anxious, fearful	0.56	**	79	B_2
69	Elated/euphoric	0.62	**	92	A
70	Moody, irritable/dysphoric	0.20		75	C
71	Suspicious/hostile	0.09		69	C
72	Tense	0.03		69	C
73	Inner restlessness	0.65	**	83	A
74	Full of complaints	0.19		88	D_2
75	Silly; fatuous	0.88	**	98	A
76	Ecstatic				D_3
77	Feeling of insufficiency, inadequacy	0.65	**	83	A
78	Exaggerated self-confidence	0.78	**	96	A
79	Guilt feelings	0.74	**	88	A
80	Feelings of impoverishment	0.66		98	D_1
81	Ambivalent	0.09		69	C
82	Inadequate affect	0.59	**	81	B_1
83	Emotional lability	–0.04		92	D_2
84	Emotional incontinence				D_3
85	Emotional rigidity	0.34	**	75	C
86	Other disturbances				D_3
Psychomotor disorders					
87	Lack of initiative and spontaneity	0.64	**	83	A
88	Inhibition of drive	0.37	**	75	C
89	Stuporous	–0.03		94	D_2
90	Mute	0.11		83	D_2
91	Exaggerated initiative and spontaneity	0.34		88	D_2
92	Motor restlessness	0.18		71	C
93	'Parakinesis'/stereotypy	0.24		90	D_2
94	Negativism				D_3
95	Mannerisms	0.19		88	D_2

Table X. AMP symptoms (contd.)

Item No.	Item	Kappa	Significant	Agreement	Category
96	Disorganized speech/neologism				D_3
97	Logorrhea	0.51	**	88	B_1
98	Other disturbances			98	D_3
Special features of course of disease					
99	Better in the evenings	0.83	**	94	A
100	Better in the mornings				D_3
101	Exacerbations at nights	–0.04		92	D_2
102	Other particularities			96	D_3
Disorders of drive and social behavior need for special care					
103	Reduced contact	0.33	*	83	D_2
104	Increased contact	0.66		98	D_1
105	Feeling of being ill	0.33	**	67	C
106	Lack of feeling of being ill	0.55	**	79	B_2
107	Lack of insight into the illness	0.54	**	77	B_2
108	Refusal of treatment	0.13		71	C
109	Suicidal tendencies	0.83	**	92	A
110	Suicidal acts	–0.03		94	D_2
111	Self-mutilation (tendency)	0.48		96	D_1
112	Aggressive tendencies	0.85	**	98	A
113	Aggressive behavior	–0.02		96	D_2
114	Increased sexual drive	0.66		98	D_1
115	Decreased sexual drive	0.96	**	98	A
116	Sexual perversions				D_3
117	Refusal to eat				D_3
118	Patient has to be fed				D_3
119	Patient has to be taken care of regarding personal hygiene				D_3
120	Incontinent of urine and feces				D_3
121	Difficult to engage in an occupation	0.19		65	C
122	Confined to bed			98	D_3
123	Other disturbances				D_3
Sleep disorders					
124	Difficulty falling asleep	0.75	**	88	A
125	Interrupted sleep	0.81	**	92	A
126	Only able to sleep for short periods	0.91	**	96	A

Table X. AMP symptoms (contd.)

Item No.	Item	Kappa	Significant	Agreement	Category
127	Drowsiness during the day	0.46		92	D_1
128	Tiredness	0.30	**	65	C
129	Increased dreaming	0.54	*	94	B_1
130	Others				D_3
Appetite disorders					
131	Decreased appetite	0.91	**	96	A
132	Increased appetite	0.65	**	96	A
133	Increased thirst	0.31		92	D_2
134	Others			98	D_3
Autonomic symptoms					
135	Nasal congestion				D_3
136	Increased salivation			98	D_3
137	Dry mouth	0.74	**	88	A
138	Seborrhea			98	D_3
139	Blurred vision	1.00	*	100	A
140	Nausea	0.56	**	92	B_1
141	Vomiting	1.00	**	100	A
142	Constipation	0.76	**	90	A
143	Diarrhea	0.79	**	98	A
144	Difficulty in urinating	0.65	**	96	A
145	Hot flashes	0.41	*	90	B_1
146	Chills	0.70	**	90	A
147	Flush				D_3
148	Sweating	0.81	**	92	A
149	Respiratory disturbances	0.24		90	D_2
150	Headache: 'pressure'	0.62	**	88	A
151	Palpitations	0.47	**	80	B_1
152	Dizziness	0.54	**	85	B_1
153	Fainting	1.00	*	100	A
154	Others			96	D_3
Additional physical symptoms					
155	Edema	1.00	*	100	A
156	Circulation related symptoms, e.g. myocardial infarction			98	D_3
157	Thrombosis-thrombophlebitis				D_3
158	Embolism				D_3
159	Galactorrhea				D_3
160	Menstrual disturbances			98	D_3
161	Local complications of injection				D_3

Table X. AMP symptoms (contd.)

Item No.	Item	Kappa	Significant	Agreement	Category
162	Pruritus				D_3
163	Photosensivity				D_3
164	Parasthesias				D_3
165	Exanthemas				D_3
166	Icterus				D_3
167	Others				D_3
Neurological symptoms					
168	Increased muscle tone			98	D_3
169	Lowered muscle tone				D_3
170	Fine tremor	0.57	**	79	B_2
171	Medium or gross tremor	–0.09		83	D_2
172	Nystagmus				D_3
173	Paroxysmal dyskinesia	0.48		96	D_1
174	Persistent hyperkinesia	–0.02		96	D_2
175	Hypokinesia	0.36	**	69	C
176	Pareses				D_3
177	Signs of the pyramidal tract				D_3
178	Ataxia				D_3
179	Other neurological symptoms				D_3
180	Akathesia			98	D_3
181	Primitive reflexes				D_3

* $p \leq 0.1$; ** $p \leq 0.05$

Table XI. AMDP symptoms

Item No.	Item	Kappa	Significant	Agreement	Category
Disorders of consciousness					
1	Lowered vigilance				D_3
2	Clouded consciousness			96	D_3
3	Narrowed consciousness				D_3
4	Expanded consciousness				D_3
Disturbances of orientation					
5	Time	0.81	**	96	A
6	Place				D_3
7	Situation				D_3
8	Self				D_3

Table XI. AMDP symptoms (contd.)

Item No.	Item	Kappa	Significant	Agreement	Category
Disturbances of attention and memory					
9	Apperception	0.54	*	94	B_1
10	Concentration	0.22		77	C
11	Memorization	0.46	*	92	B_1
12	Retention	0.33	**	69	C
13	Confabulation				D_3
14	Paramnesias			98	D_3
Formal disorders of thought					
15	Inhibited thinking	0.48	**	77	B_2
16	Retarded thinking	0.62	**	81	A
17	Circumstantial thinking	0.08		71	C
18	Restricted thinking	0.54	**	77	B_2
19	Perseveration	–0.04		92	D_2
20	Rumination	0.66	**	83	A
21	Pressured thinking	–0.08		85	D_2
22	Flight of ideas	0.34		87	D_2
23	Tangential thinking	0.50	**	79	B_2
24	Blocking	0.34	**	69	C
25	Incoherence	0.40	**	83	B_1
26	Neologisms				D_3
Phobias and compulsions					
27	Suspiciousness	–0.09		83	D_2
28	Hypochondriasis			98	D_3
29	Phobias				D_3
30	Obsessive thoughts	0.37		94	D_2
31	Compulsive impulses	–0.02		96	D_2
32	Compulsive actions			98	D_3
Delusions					
33	Delusional mood	0.75	**	88	A
34	Delusional perceptions	–0.03		73	C
35 36	Sudden delusional idea Delusional ideas	0.52	**	77	B_2
37	Systematized delusions	0.65	**	88	A
38	Delusional dynamics	0.50	**	79	B_2
39	Delusions of reference	0.52	**	79	B_2
40	Delusions of persecution	0.66	**	83	A
41	Delusions of jealousy				D_3
42	Delusions of guilt	0.26		90	D_2
43	Delusions of impoverishment			98	D_3
44	Hypochondriac delusions				D_3

Table XI. AMDP symptoms (contd.)

Item No.	Item	Kappa	Significant	Agreement	Category
45	Delusions of grandeur	0.81	**	96	A
46	Other delusions			90	D_3
Disorders of perception					
47	Illusions			94	D_3
48	Verbal (phonemic) hallucinations	0.89	**	96	A
49	Other auditory hallucinations	1.00	**	100	A
50	Visual hallucinations	0.65	**	96	A
51	Bodily hallucinations (coenesthetic)	0.55	**	88	B_1
52	Olfactory or gustatory halluzinations	1.00	*	100	A
Disorders of ego					
53	Derealization	0.19		88	D_2
54	Depersonalization	0.61	**	90	A
55	Thought broadcasting	0.56	**	84	B_1
56	Thought withdrawal	–0.03		90	D_2
57	Thought insertion	0.56	**	83	B_1
58	Other feelings of alien influence	0.33	**	77	C
Disturbances of affect					
59	Perplexity	0.41	**	81	B_1
60	Feeling of loss of feeling	0.48	**	77	B_2
61	Blunted affect	0.13		58	C
62	Felt loss of vitality	0.49	**	75	B_2
63	Depressed mood	0.95	**	98	A
64	Hopelessness	0.62	**	81	A
65	Anxiety	0.52	**	77	B_2
66	Euphoria	0.73	**	94	A
67	Dysphoria	0.19		69	C
68	Irritability				
69	Inner restlessness	0.61	**	81	A
70	Complaintiveness	0.15		85	D_2
71	Feelings of inadequacy	0.58	**	81	B_1
72	Exaggerated self-esteem	0.88	**	98	A
73	Feelings of guilt	0.74	**	88	A
74	Feelings of impoverishment	0.66		98	D_1
75	Ambivalence	0.09		69	C
76	Parathymia	0.63	**	83	A

Table XI. AMDP symptoms (contd.)

Item No.	Item	Kappa	Significant	Agreement	Category
77	Affective lability	–0.04		92	D_2
78	Affective incontinence				D_3
79	Affective rigidity	0.37	**	77	C
Disorders of drive and psychomotility					
80	Lack of drive	0.60	**	81	A
81	Inhibition of drive	0.43	**	77	B_2
82	Increased drive	0.34		88	D_2
83	Motor restlessness	–0.01		67	C
84	Parakinesia	0.18		88	D_2
85	Mannerisms	0.39		90	D_2
86	Histrionics	–0.02		96	D_2
87	Mutism	0.11		83	D_2
88	Logorrhea	0.51	**	88	B_1
Circadian disturbances					
89	Worse in the morning	0.83	**	94	A
90	Worse in the evening				
91	Better in the evening				D_3
Other disturbances					
92	Social withdrawal	0.29		81	D_2
93	Excessive social contact	0.66		98	D_1
94	Aggressiveness	0.66		98	D_1
95	Suicidal tendencies	0.79	**	90	A
96	Self-mutilation	0.66		98	D_1
97	Lack of feeling ill	0.60	**	81	A
98	Lack of insight	0.50	**	75	B_2
99	Uncooperativeness	0.15		73	C
100	Lack of self-care				D_3
Disturbances of sleep and vigilance					
101	Difficulty falling asleep (early insomnia)	0.75	**	88	A
102	Interrupted sleep (middle insomnia)	0.81	**	92	A
103	Shortened sleep	0.87	**	94	A
104	Early waking (late insomnia)	0.70	**	90	A
105	Drowsiness	0.21	*	60	C
Appetite disturbances					
106	Decreased appetite	0.91	**	96	A
107	Excessive appetite	0.65	**	96	A

Table XI. AMDP symptoms (comtd.)

Item No.	Item	Kappa	Significant	Agreement	Category
108	Excessive thirst	0.54	*	94	B_1
109	Decreased libido	0.62	**	81	A
Gastrointestinal disturbances					
110	Hypersalivation			98	D_3
111	Dry mouth	0.69	**	85	A
112	Nausea	0.47	*	92	B_1
113	Vomiting	1.00	**	100	A
114	Gastric discomfort	–0.04		88	D_2
115	Constipation	0.76	**	90	A
116	Diarrhea				
Cardiac-respiratory disturbances					
117	Breathing difficulties	0.29		92	D_2
118	Dizziness	0.54	**	86	B_1
119	Palpitations	0.70	**	88	A
120	Cardiac pain				
Other autonomic disturbances					
121	Blurred vision	1.00	*	100	A
122	Increased perspiration	0.81	**	92	A
123	Seborrhea				D_3
124	Micturition difficulties	0.65	**	96	A
125	Menstrual disturbances			98	D_3
Other somatic disturbances					
126	Headache	0.62	**	88	A
127	Backache	1.00	*	100	A
128	Heaviness in the legs	–0.03		90	D_2
129	Hot flashes	0.41	*	90	B_1
130	Chills	0.70	**	90	A
131	Conversion symptoms			98	D_3
Neurological disturbances					
132	Hypertonia				D_3
133	Hypotonia			98	D_3
134	Tremor	0.83	**	92	A
135	Acute dyskinesia	0.65	**	96	A
136	Hypokinesia	0.43	**	73	B_2
137	Akathisia			98	D_3
138	Ataxia				D_3
139	Nystagmus				D_3
140	Paresthesia				D_3

$* P \leq 0.1$; $** P \leq 0.05$.

Conclusions

Our study shows a good interrater reliability for symptoms of the AMP and AMDP-Systems. Thanks to a more precise description, the AMDP items have an interrater reliability which is slightly better than the one of the AMP items.

References

Angst, J.; Battegay, R.; Bente, D.; Berner, P.; Broeren, W.; Cornu, F.; Dick, P.; Engelmeier, M.-P.; Heimann, H.; Heinrich, K.; Helmchen, H.; Hippius, H.; Poeldinger, W.; Schmiedlin, P.; Schmitt, W.; Weis, P.: Das Dokumentationssystem der Arbeitsgemeinschaft für Methodik und Dokumentation in der Psychiatrie (AMP). Arzneimittel- Forsch. *19:* 339–405 (1969).

Cohen J.: A coefficient of agreement for nominal scales. Educ. Psychol. Measmt *20:* 37–46 (1960).

Cohen, J.: Weighted chi square: an extension of the kappa method. Educ. Psychol. Measmt *32:* 61–74 (1972).

Everitt, B. C.: Moments of the statistics kappa and weighted kappa. Br. J. math. statist. Psychol. *21:* 97–103 (1968).

Fleiss, J. L.; Cohen, J.; Everitt, B. S.: Large sample standard errors of kappa and weighted kappa. Psychol. Bull.. *72:* 323–327 (1969).

Guy, W.; Ban, T. A.: The AMDP-system (Springer, Berlin 1982).

Helmchen, H.: The AMP system as a method in clinical pharmacopsychiatry; Assessment of pharmacodynamic effects in human pharmacology. I. Psychopharmacological screening tests (Schattauer, Stuttgart 1975).

Langer, F.; Schulz von Thun, F.: Messung komplexer Merkmale in Psychologie und Pädagogik (Reinhardt, München 1974).

Scharfetter, C.: Das AMP-System. Manual. 2. Aufl. (Springer, Berlin 1972).

Tinsley, H. E. A.; Weiss, D. J.: Interrater reliability and agreement of subjective judgment. J. Counseling Psychol. *22:* 358–376 (1975).

Woggon, B.; Baumann, U.; Angst, J.: Interrater-Reliabilität von AMP-Symptomen. Arch. Psychiat. Nervenkrankh. *225: 73–85* (1978).

S. Kuny, MD, Research Department, Psychiatric University Hospital, PO Box 68, CH-8029 Zürich (Switzerland)

Mod. Probl. Pharmacopsychiat., vol. 20, pp. 161–173 (Karger, Basel 1983)

Interrater Reliability of the French AMDP Psychopathology Scale: A New Measurement in Single Cases

D. Bobon, R. von Frenckell, C. Mormont

Department of Psychiatry, University of Liège Medical School, Liège, Belgium

The first edition of the Manual by the Association for Methodology and Documentation in Psychiatry AMDP [*Bobon*, 1978] was a partial and provisional adaptation of the system; it did not include its anamnestic sheets, and the psychopathological as well as the somatic scales were based on the February 1977 Vienna draft of the German revision, since this revision was still in preparation when the French manuscript went into print. The French manual was considered as a sort of 'zero edition' aimed at collecting empirical information on the difficulties encountered by French-speaking psychiatrists and psychologists rating psychopathology on the basis of German concepts and their AMDP codification.

Besides a very close interaction between the French and German revision groups [*Bobon*, this volume], the former made a wide use of video sessions to test the feasibility and the interrater reliability of the AMDP Psychopathology Scale. A total of 207 videotaped interviews were evaluated in our department, while 9 selected interviews were circulated and rated at various meetings of the French-speaking AMDP section. Thanks to such an intensive research, the French revision of the manual [*Bobon*, 1981] is not only fully compatible with the German revision [Arbeitsgemeinschaft für Methodik und Dokumentation in der Psychiatrie, 1979, 1981] but it eliminates or stresses the pitfalls for French-speaking raters and the few divergences with the German manual.

The aim of the studies summarized here was to analyze the interrater reliability (IRR) of groups of raters who would be as heterogeneous as possible from the standpoint of their mother tongue, psychiatric education and AMDP training. Therefore, a limited number of videotapes were projected to different raters on several occasions.

Difficulties arose with the statistical analysis of such data. As discussed by *von Frenckell and Bobon* [1982], all known methods necessitate either dichotomous ratings or more patients than raters; all of them are univariate applications, including the recent a_2 pairwise agreement ratio [*Busch* et al., 1980, 1981; *Renfordt* et al., this volume]. As for the kappa coefficient, it has serious limitations which are admitted by the very authors who use it [*Woggon* et al., 1978; *Baumann and Woggon,* 1979]. Moreover, these methods do not allow a visualization of the global distances between raters.

For these reasons, we turned to a classical technique, namely, the obverse factor analysis or Q-technique. As we will see, the two-factor solution gives a satisfactory approach to the visualization of the rating patterns. The multivariate indexes of variance calculated by the factor analysis (FA) program for each item and for each factor – the factor scores (FS) and generalized distances D^2 – were used as a measure of IRR. Several videotaped patients have been analyzed and reported according to this method [*von Frenckell* et al., 1979; *Mirel* et al., 1980; *Bobon and Dufour,* 1982; *Bobon and Pichot,* 1982].

By adding new raters to these cases and reanalyzing our data, we came across two biases in the application of FA to the measurement of IRR. Firstly, despite a similar standard deviation, an item with a high mean value tended to have a high FS while an item with a low mean tended to have a low FS. Secondly, items for which all raters agree on the same severity have FS differing from zero.

With help of simulated ratings, the influence of $\overline{X}$ on FS was confirmed and the FA program was modified to locate a zero dispersion at the origin of the FS [*von Frenckell and Bobon,* 1982].

Subject and Method

Patient. Mrs. FER. is a 36-year-old housekeeper from Marseille. She was hospitalized for the first time when she was 17 with the diagnosis of delusional mania. In 18 years, she was readmitted seven times for episodes of incoherence, parathymia, delusions of grandeur, fantasy and persecution. From one episode to the other, her mood was swinging from mania to suicidal tendencies.

She was videotaped in a delusional manic phase in the CCTV studio of the Department of Psychiatry in Marseille by Dr. *D. Pringuey,* a trained AMDP psychiatrist. Her strong accent and a volubile speech contributed to the difficulties encountered by some participants in evaluating the patient, but she was selected for the present analysis because she illustrates several basic aspects of comparative psychiatry and because she has been documented by the most representative sample of French-speaking raters.

Video. The interview was free. The camera was not concealed. The patient's name was not mentioned during the interview and the projections of the recording were strictly limited to the participants to rating sessions.

The recording was evaluated on five occasions: 'pilot ratings' in the Psychiatric Departments of Liège and Marseille (April 1979), 11th International Meeting of the French-Speaking AMDP Section (St-Maximin/Marseille, April 1979), Annual Training Weekend in our department (November 1979), 'Canadian Projection' at the tristandard CCTV studio of the Union Chimique Belge (Brussels, March 1981).

A first analysis of IRR was undertaken after the two 'pilot ratings' and its results reported at the next session, the St-Maximin International Meeting. Being aware of the main divergences between the pilot raters, the audience evaluated or reevaluated the videotape. After the participants had individually rated the patient, a discussion moderated by an AMDP specialist took place and ended in a 'consensus score' for each item.

Raters. The four 1979 sessions, evaluated by means of the first edition of the AMDP Scale, totalled 58 participants from ten countries: France (28 raters), Belgium (18), Austria and Germany (4), Algeria (2), French-speaking Switzerland (2), Greece, Luxemburg, Portugal and Spain (1 each). The 1981 session, evaluated by means of the revised scale, was attended by 15 participants, all Belgians except for one Algerian psychiatrist postgraduating in Liège. Raters who evaluated at least two projections will be referred to as TR raters (test-retest). The consensus ratings are included in the analyses in order to study their relationship with the individual ratings.

Table I indicates the average training in general psychopathology and in the AMDP Scale as estimated by the participants themselves on a 5-point scale. For the sake of brevity, the results of the retest ratings and of the only session evaluated with the revision of the AMDP will not be analyzed but briefly mentioned whenever pertinent.

Table I. Mean training in general psychopathology and in the AMDP Psychopathology Scale of all participants who rated FER for the first time with the first edition (T = test) and for the subgroup who rated the patient on two occasions (TR = test-retest). In brackets, the number of participants who filled out the 5-point self-rating on their training as compared to the total number of raters included in the analyses

	T (n = 56 : 58)	TR (n = 14 : 15)
Psychopathology	2.68 ± 0.94	2.86 ± 0.66
AMDP scale	1.45 ± 1.17	2.50 ± 0.65

Ratings. The 1979 projections were documented on the basis of the first edition of the AMDP Psychopathology Scale [*Bobon,* 1978], which comprises 122 items graduated from 0 to 4: absent-slight-moderate-severe-very severe (in the English and French versions of the AMDP Scales, this range has been given the preference over the German 0–3 range for three reasons: clinical need of two categories instead of one in severe cases, greater sensitivity of item scores, less central tendency).

Each participant filled out an identification card (IC) bearing his name, sex, mother tongue, main place of psychiatric training, and self-evaluation of his familiarity with general psychopathology as well as with the AMDP (on a 5-point scale: nil-poor-medium-good-excellent). The IC also beared the approval versus refusal of the rater to eventually mention his name in reporting results.

Statistical Analyses. In a first step (fig. 1), we applied the standard BMDP4M program of principal components FA [*Dixon,* 1981]; in order to calculate the correlation coefficients between raters, we performed an obverse FA according to the Q-technique by substituting the individuals (i.e. the raters) for the variables (i.e. the items).

In the second step, illustrated by figures 2 and 3, we substracted the mean value of item scores with help of an ad hoc program before performing the BMDP4M and we made use of the OCORR option of this program in order to compute the factor scores FS from the origin, thus eliminating the two biases introduced by the application of the standard FA to the calculation of IRR [for methodological details, see *von Frenckell and Bobon,* 1982]. A rotation was not performed.

Several arbitrary selection criteria were used. For determining the number of factors to be analyzed, *Grelet* et al. [not dated] recommend the

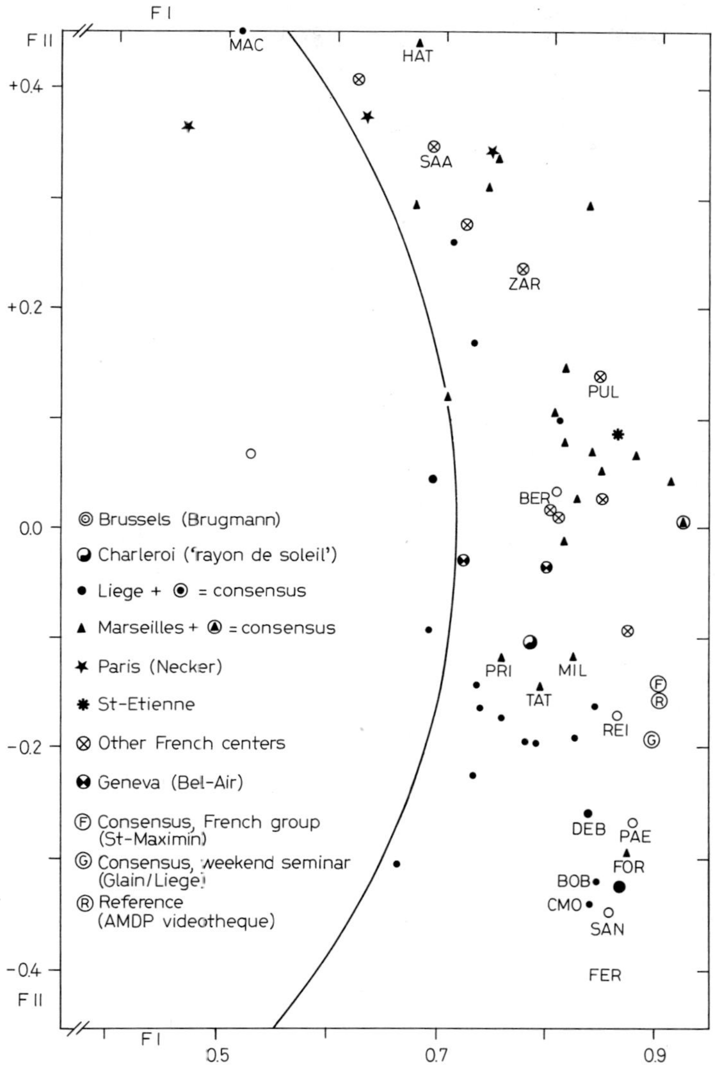

Fig. 1. Loadings of the 58 raters and 4 consensuses in the first two factors of the standard FA. Arc of circle = loading of 0.700 = h^2 of 0.50. O Other countries.

relative difference between latent roots. In the standard two-factor solution, a communality h^2 of 0.50 is a convenient threshold to determine whether a rater's variance is well enough represented in this solution or not. In the modified FA, a loading of 0.500 usually selects, in our experience, a sufficient number of 'extreme' raters at each factor pole.

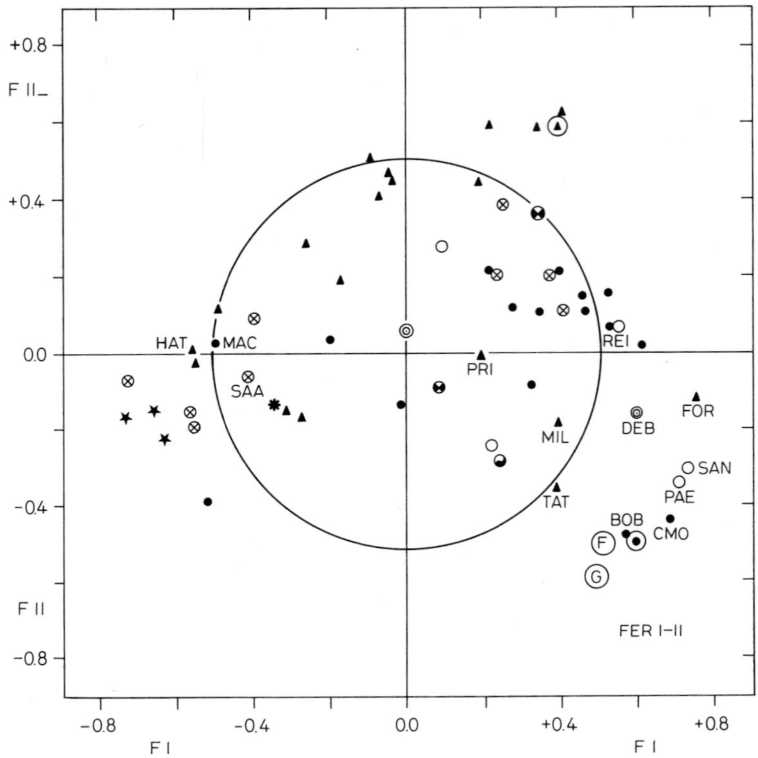

Fig. 2. Same data as figure 1 with the modified FA. Circle = loading of 0.500 (see Method).

Results and Discussion

Table II gives the percentages of variance explained by the first five factors for the standard versus the modified FA. The criterion of the relative difference between latent roots indicates that factor IV is the last in the standard FA which adds a notable percentage of variance to the preceding factor (as compared to seven factors according to the Kaiser criterion); in the modified FA, the relative difference becomes small after factor III.

In a previous analysis of the first 44 raters [*Mirel* et al., 1980], we had applied the standard FA. The inclusion of new raters completes but does not alter the initial picture (fig. 1). The small number of raters falling un-

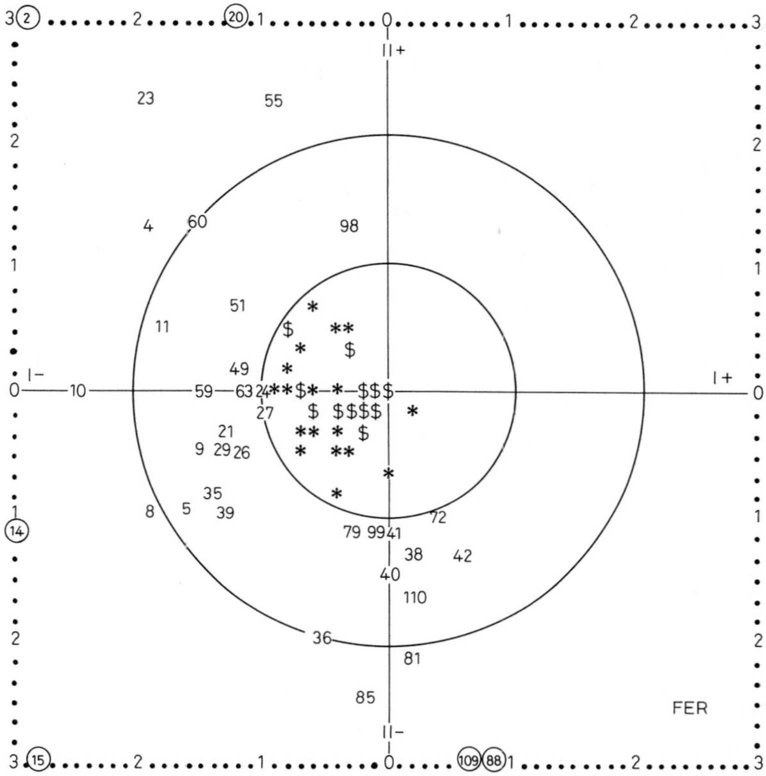

Fig. 3. Factor scores of the 122 psychopathological items in the first two factors of the modified FA. FS < 1.000 (inner circle) = asterisks and dollar signs; FS ≥ 1.000 versus 2.000 (outer circle) = item number. Items on the frame are encircled to avoid misinterpretation.

der the arbitrary communality threshold of 0.50 indicates that the first two factors of the standard FA give a fair estimate of the variance.

The first factor of the standard FA explains 62% of the total variance; in this unipolar factor, all raters have a positive and mostly high loading. F_{II} explains only 5% of the variance but it stretches the raters along a bipolar axis. Globally, the raters opposed in the standard F_{II} are the same as the raters opposed in the modified F_I (fig. 2); the only major difference lies in a sign inversion. This illustrates the fact that the suppression of the mean value of the item scores is responsible for the disappearance of the first standard factor, confirmed by the difference in the number of factors retained before and after this modification of FA. This operation corresponds approximately to the elimination of the items 'absent' since the comparison of the two opposite consensuses (Liège and Marseille) shows that, if both ratings agree on 90 items, 86 of these items are 'absent'.

The average training of the extreme raters of the first two modified factors is given in table III (the last factor – standard F_{IV}, modified F_{III} – will not be analyzed in the present paper; it contrasts Belgian postgraduate students with French senior psychiatrists who share poor skills in AMDP rating).

Table III and its comparison with table I shows that the raters of the positive pole of the modified F_I (fig. 2), corresponding to the negative pole of the standard F_{II} (fig. 1) have the best experience in psychopathology and a better AMDP training than the raters of the opposite pole, who have a good psychopathological experience but a poor AMDP one.

Figure 2 further reveals that the highest loadings of F_{I+} correspond to: (a) the two French-speaking participants who have the longest and the most intensive experience with the AMDP-System, namely the psychiatrist *Bobon* (BOB) and the psychologist *Mormont* (CMO) from Liège; (b) three of the four consensuses: the one reached in Liège after the pilot rating, as well as both international ones; (c) two senior psychiatrists who had never met and who rated on two different occasions but who shared an excellent knowledge of German psychopathology and of the AMDP-System: the Portuguese *Paes de Sousa* (PAE) and the Spaniard *Sanchez Blanque* (SAN); (d) farther away from this core, three raters with various trainings: the Belgian *De Buck* (DEB), the Frenchman *Fornari* (FOR) and the German *Rein* (REI).

The Marseille collaborators with a greater psychopathological *and* AMDP experience are closest to the core: *Tatossian* (TAT), who recently succeeded to *Sutter* as professor of psychiatry in Marseille and who has an outstanding knowledge of the German psychopathological-phenomenological literature, and a German postgraduating in Marseille, *Milech* (MIL). A third collaborator, the interviewer *Pringuey* (PRI), trained by *Tatossian,* is close to him in figure 1 but figure 2 reveals that PRI actually has a rating pattern different from the raters of F_I and F_{II}, his correlation with both these factors being very low.

The participants determining the opposite pole (F_{II+} in fig. 1, F_{I-} in fig. 2) are French raters from various centers, a senior psychologist of Al-

Table II. Latent roots (Eigenvalues EV), relative differences between these values (Δ), percentage of the total variance (% V) and cumulative variance (cum. V) of the first 5 factors before and after modifications of the method; n = 58 T raters

	Standard FA				Modified FA			
	EV	Δ	% V	cum. V	EV	Δ	% V	cum. V
I	38.17	0.92	61.57	61.57	12.06	0.55	19.46	19.46
II	3.06	0.39	4.94	66.51	5.47	0.23	8.83	28.28
III	1.87	0.05	3.01	69.52	4.24	0.30	6.83	35.12
IV	1.78	0.34	2.87	72.39	2.96	0.14	4.78	39.90
V	1.18	0.06	1.90	74.29	2.56	0.07	4.12	44.01

Table III. Mean training in general psychopathology and in the AMDP Psychopathology Scale for the raters whose loading in the modified F_I and/or F_{II} is ⩾ 0.500 (0.350 in the case of F_{II}.)

	F_I		F_{II}	
	⊖ (n = 10)	⊕ (n = 10)	⊖ (n = 4)	⊕ (n = 3)
Psychopathology	2.50 ± 0.71	2.90 ± 1.20	3.00 ± 1.41	3.00 ± 0.00
AMDP scale	0.80 ± 0.63	2.10 ± 1.45	2.00 ± 1.83	2.00 ± 0.00

Table IV. Frequency distribution of the degrees of severity, mean and standard deviation for items 14 (confabulation) and 15 (paramnesias) for the extreme raters of each pole of factor I, for these raters as a whole and for all raters, including 4 consensuses. NA = Not ascertained; AB = absent; MI = mild; MO = moderate; SV = severe; EX = extremely severe

Factor	n	NA	AB	MI	MO	SV	EX	$\bar{X}$ ± s
Confabulation								
I−	10	0	0	0	0	3	7	3.70 ± 0.48
I+	12	0	12	0	0	0	0	0.00 ± 0.00
I total	22	0	12	0	0	3	7	1.68 ± 1.91
All	62		44	1	1	6	10	0.98 ± 1.61
Paramnesias								
I−	10	0	0	0	0	4	6	3.60 ± 0.52
I+	12	3	8	0	0	1	0	0.25 ± 0.87
I total	22	3	8	0	0	5	6	1.77 ± 1.85
All	62		37	0	3	13	9	1.31 ± 1.65

gerian origin, *Saadi* (SAA), a Greek psychiatrist postgraduating in Marseille, *Hatziagorou* (HAT), and an Algerian psychiatrist postgraduating in Liège, (MAC). The proximity of these three participants, who rated during different sessions and never met, illustrates a rating pattern developed below.

The second modified factor (fig. 2) opposes the core raters to a group of raters from Marseille who have lower loadings in F_I, except for their consensus and its moderator. It is noteworthy that these contrasted participants have a comparable insight in psychopathology and AMDP (table III).

In other words, F_I seems to be influenced by AMDP training in the main place, F_{II} by different schools rather than different durations of psychiatric training.

All consensuses except one are close to the most experienced raters, including participants from Marseille who are used to evaluate pathology in the patient's culture. The so-called reference rating (R in fig. 1), established by us on the basis of the consensuses and of individual ratings by experienced participants, may be considered as an optimal symptom profile.

How about the items responsible for the interrater disagreements?

According to the simulation studies by *von Frenckell and Bobon* [1982], figure 3 may be interpreted as follows: (1) the more a FS is distant from the origin of a factor, the more the raters responsible for this factor disagree on the item score; (2) the farther a FS from the origin, the higher the score given to the item by the raters with the same sign.

Moreover, since there is an intrinsic relationship between rater axes (fig. 2) and item axes (fig. 3), the latter figure does not only visualize FS coordinates in two factors but it also permits 'causal' interpretations on IRR. For example, the bad IRR of item 10 on disorders of apperception is specifically due to the F_I raters, i.e. to AMDP training; this interpretation is confirmed by the results of retest (FS from 1.683 down to 0.545 in the TR subgroup), and of the second edition (FS = 0.916).

But these figures do not indicate the magnitude of dispersion at the respective rater poles. As stated above, the sign of a FS does not point to its standard deviation but to its mean value. The modified FA has to be complemented with a frequency distribution for the extreme raters of each pole, an arbitrary value being attributed to the loadings in order to select a sufficient number of raters at each pole. An application of this procedure to items 14 and 15 (table IV) demonstrates that almost identical FS values may conceal quite different dispersions: (a) in the case of item 14, the raters with the same sign as the FS have the higher $\overline{X}$ and the higher SD; (b) in the case of item 15, the higher $\overline{X}$ characterizes the raters with the same sign but the higher SD characterizes the opposite raters.

Figure 2 further indicates that item 14 (confabulation) and item 15 (paramnesias) have a bad IRR related to the AMDP trained versus untrained raters of F_I and, as regards item 15, to equally trained raters of F_{II}.

Confabulation has a much higher FS on F_I than on F_{II}, reflecting the fact that its bad IRR is due to the French raters of F_{I-} rather than to the Marseilles raters of F_{II+}. This corresponds altogether to an insufficient training in the AMDP terminology and to a characteristic of French psychiatry, which ignores to a large extent the difference made in German-speaking countries between fabulation and confabulation.

Paramnesias (including delusional memories) have a low IRR in both factors. All the AMDP-untrained raters of F_{I-} rate the symptom as severe or very severe (table IV), whereas most experienced raters of F_{I+} consider that the patient has phantasies which differ from delusional memories but three of them give a 'doubtful' answer; the largest consensus (St-Maximin) rate it 'severe'! We explain this indecision partly by deficiencies in the manual, in which the difference between delusional memories and sudden delusional ideas is not operational enough. The low IRR on the second factor reflects deep conceptual disagreements: all F_{II+} raters, who are with the Department of Psychiatry in Marseille, evaluate delusional memories as absent in agreement with all non-Marseille raters from F_{II-} but in contradiction with the two experienced Marseille raters of this pole, *Milech* and *Tatossian,* who rate them as severe versus very severe.

Before concluding, one should mention that statistical analyses do not replace a careful descriptive analysis of data. The comparison of the two opposite consensuses of Liège and Marseille reveals a slight but systematic difference with respect to the severity of the manic symptoms. The Liège consensus gives one more point than Marseille to delusions of grandeur, euphoria, exaggerated self-esteem, increased drive and accelerated thinking, two more points to logorrhea; this 'transcultural' difference disappears in the statistical analysis of the group at large except for exaggerated self-esteem.

Conclusion

The main reasons for a poor IRR are, according to the present study and similar ones: the video technique itself, including the interview technique – in Liège, we always use the semi-structured interview developed for the AMDP by *Bobon* et al. [1978], and revised for the second edition; psychiatric education (e.g. confabulation); AMDP training (e.g. apperception); deficiences in the manual (e.g. paramnesias); cultural thresholds (e.g. manic symptoms).

The consensus method cancels out individual failures in knowledge, AMDP training, attention span, etc.; it gives results generally close to sophisticated statistical analyses. The similarity of several consensuses reached on different occasions by different participants and different moderators raises hopes for valid and acceptable standard profiles; within the French-speaking group, this patient is in fact the first reference case of an AMDP videotheque.

The lack of operational criteria for grading the severity of symptoms might well weaken the IRR of the AMDP Scales and its sensitivity to change but it turns to a definite advantage in the case of research on the IRR itself, which constitutes a prerequise to further progress in the measurement of psychopathology at an international level.

References

Arbeitsgemeinschaft für Methodik und Dokumentation in der Psychiatrie (ed.): Das AMDP Manual, 3. Aufl. (Springer, Berlin 1979); reprinting 1981.

Baumann, U.; Woggon, B.: Interrater-Reliabilität bei Diagnosen, AMP-Syndromen und AMP-Symptomen. Arch. Psychiat. NervKrankh. *227:* 3–15 (1979).

Bobon, D. P. (ed.). Le manuel AMDP (Presses universitaires de Liège, Liège 1978).

Bobon, D. P. (ed.). Le système AMDP; 2e éd. (Mardaga, Bruxelles 1981).

Bobon, D. P.; Dufour, H.: Fidélité intercotateurs de l'échelle psychopathologique AMDP. III. Les délirants CRO et NOC évalués à l'aide de la version française révisée; in Sizaret, CR 79e Congr. Psychiat. Neurol. franç., pp. 738–744 (Masson, Paris 1982).

Bobon, D. P.; Mormont, C.; Mirel, J.: Un entretien psychopathologique semi-structuré adapté à l'échelle AMDP-3 et à l'évaluation vidéo en temps aveugle. Acta psychiat. belg. *78:* 606–618 (1978).

Bobon, D. P.; Pichot, P.: Evaluaciones mediante el sistema audiovisual de la escala psicopatologica AMDP francesa: divergencias transculturales vs. individuales. Actas luso-esp. Neurol. Psiquiat. *10*: 397–404 (1982).

Busch, H.; Cranach, M. von; Gulbinat, W.; Renfordt, E.; Tegeler, J.: Reliability of the AMDP system. A preliminary report on a multicentre exercise on the reliability of psychopathological assessment. Acta psychiat. scand. *62:* 382–392 (1980).

Busch, H.; Cranach, M. von; Gulbinat, W.; Renfordt, E.; Tegeler, J.: Methodological and practical aspects of a multicentre study of reliability of psychopathological assessment; in Sartorius, Helmchen, Multicentre trials. Mod. Probl. Pharmacopsychiat., vol. 16, pp. 37–50 (Karger, Basel 1981).

Dixon, W.J. (ed.). Biomedical computer programs, P-series (University of California Press, Berkeley 1981).

Frenckell, R. von; Berner, P.; Bobon, D.P.; Dick, P.; Dufour, H.; Heimann, H.; Huber, J.P.; Luccioni, H.; Mombour, W.; Mormont, C.; Piree, S.; Pringuey, D.; Rein, W.: Etude préliminaire de la fidélité intercotateurs de l'échelle psychopathologique AMDP; in Sizaret, CR 76e Congr. Psychiat. Neurol. franç., pp. 408–412 (Masson, Paris 1979).

Frenckell, R. von; Bobon, D.P.: L'analyse factorielle: une mesure de la fidélité intercotateurs de cas uniques. Application à l'échelle psychopathologique AMDP. Acta psychiat. belg. *82:* 117–135 (1982).

Grelet, Y.; Jambu, M.; Lebeaux, M.D.: Exemples de sorties de programmes. Bull. Ass. Dével. Diffus. Anal. Données, nº 6 (not dated).

Mirel, J.; Frenckell, R. von; Berner, P.; Bobon, D.P.; De Buck, R.; Dick, P.; Dufour, H.; Huber, J.P.; Luccioni, H.; Mombour, W.; Mormont, C.; Paes de Sousa, M.; Pringuey, D.; Pull, C.; Rein, W.; Sanchez Blanque, A.; Zarifian, E.: Fidélité intercotateurs de l'échelle psychopathologique AMDP. II. Distances entre cotateurs et analyse d'items d'une délirante et d'une déprimée; in Sizaret, CR 77e Congr. Psychiat. Neurol. franç., pp. 518–525 (Masson, Paris 1980).

Woggon, B.; Baumann, U.; Angst, J.: Interrater-Reliabilität von AMP-Symptomen. Arch. Psychiat. NervKrankh. *225:* 73–85 (1978).

Dr. D. Bobon, Clinique psychiatrique universitaire, 58, rue St-Laurent, B-4000 Liège (Belgique)

Mod. Probl. Pharmacopsychiat., vol. 20, pp. 174–184 (Karger, Basel 1983)

Validity of the AMP-System for Its Use in Clinical Psychopharmacology

J. Angst, B. Woggon

Psychiatric University Hospital Zürich, Research Department, Zürich, Switzerland

Introduction

This paper is based on 13 years of experience with the AMP (Arbeitsgemeinschaft für Methodik und Dokumentation in der Psychiatrie) system, including 58 drug trials performed between 1967 and 1980. We use the name AMP-System instead of AMDP-System, because our data were collected while the first version of the AMP-System was still used. This paper does not deal with the validity of the AMP-System in general, but with its validity for the use in clinical psychopharmacology. According to *Carmines and Zeller* [1979] one cannot validate an instrument itself, but validate the instrument in relation to the purpose for which it is being used. We shall concentrate on two aspects of the validity: (1) content validity and (2) criterion-related validity.

As *content validity* we understand the extent to which a rating scale represents aspects about the present state of a patient which are relevant in psychopharmacology for the measurement of change. But what does 'measurement of change' mean? It means quantitative and qualitative changes of symptoms and side effects, i.e., it should reflect the most important changes of the clinical picture occurring during a psychopharmacological treatment.

Drugs cannot only quantitatively improve or deteriorate a psychopathological condition, they may also induce important qualitative changes. These changes cover a wide spectrum of clinical symptoms and, therefore, require a very comprehensive inventory of characteristics to assess them.

Let us give some examples: treatment is started in a depressed patient. During this treatment the depression is gradually diminishing and changes to a mixed state of manic and depressive symptoms. Finally it even switches to hypomania or mania. In other cases – especially when applying anticholinergic tricyclic or tetracyclic antidepressants – the depression may transitorily change to a confusional state with disorientation of time and space and, finally, to a toxic delirious state with illusions, hallucinations, anxiety, agitation, and severe tremor. When applying neuroleptic drugs in schizophrenic or other psychotic patients, similar dramatic qualitative changes of the symptomatology may occur, like confusional states, or the clinical picture may be changing from an acute paranoid hallucinatory state with excitation to stupor and – after weeks or months – into a classical depression or mania. In other cases the patient may develop severe and persistent neurological side effects requiring a careful assessment. These examples already show how complex and elaborate the inventory for measuring changes during drug trials should be if we really intend to measure what occurs empirically and not only certain aspects of drug action. Usually this problem is dealt with by applying different types of instruments, especially designed for measuring special changes, e.g., depression and mania, neurological and other side effects. In many cases it is very difficult and arbitrary to distinguish between effects and side effects. If, e.g., a depression changes into hypomania, is this change considered to be drug induced or is it a spontaneous change as in bipolar disorder? Should it, therefore, not be assessed by an instrument measuring both mania and depression? This switch occurs in about 5% of all antidepressant treatments. It is very similar in the field of the so-called side effects, e.g., dryness of the mouth may be as well a symptom of anxiety and tension as a symptom of an anticholinergic action of the drug. How should we be able to distinguish between symptoms and side effects in such a case? A third example concerns tardive dyskinesia. The oral dyskinetic movements have been observed not only as a side effect of drugs, but as a spontaneous phenomenon in elderly patients, too. How should we distinguish the two types, if they are clinically identical? Should we not include these phenomena as ordinary symptoms of a possible clinical picture into the inventory of items of our rating scales in order to avoid to overlook them systematically?

Again, these few examples show that it is a questionable procedure to generally start with highly specific instruments for measuring changes. Of course, choosing specific instruments with a narrow scope of meas-

Table I: Clinical syndromes represented by five rating scales

Clinical syndromes	HAMD	BPRS	CPRS	IMPS	AMP
Schizophrenia		+	+	+	+
Depression	+	+	+	+	+
Mania			+	+	+
Organic psychoses				+	+
Neuroses					+
Side effects			+		+

urement may have high validity in a certain field, e.g., measuring the antidepressant action, and it may also have a high reliability. But we may also lose a lot of information on events occurring during the treatment in the field of unexpected changes and side effects. Research of today has no more the task just to assess whether a drug is antipsychotic or antidepressant, but it should specify as detailed as possible the differential action of drugs in terms of effects and side effects. For this purpose we need more complex instruments. The content of some well-known rating scales is listed in table I. Compared to the other scales the AMP-System covers a wider spectrum of symptoms.

Up to now only two studies dealt with the criterion-related validity, comparing the AMP-System with other rating scales. *Saarma and Morozov* [1978] found a slightly higher sensitivity of the AMP Scales measuring changes during a drug treatment of depression and schizophrenia compared to the Brief Psychiatric Rating Scale (BPRS) and the Hamilton Rating Scale for Depression (HAMD total score). *Pecknold* et al. [1975] found no significant differences of the sensitivity between the AMP and the BPRS total scores during a treatment with clomacran, but significantly more changes on the level of symptoms were assessed by the AMP than by BPRS, suggesting a higher sensitivity of the AMP-System, too. In both studies [*Pecknold* et al., 1975; *Saarma and Morozov,* 1978] a direct correlation between the instruments based on scale scores was not carried out.

Based on our drug trials this section will deal with correlations between the AMP subscales and total scales and other instruments. In order to examine the criterion-related validity the syndromes of the AMP-System were correlated with the syndromes of four other rating scales. These correlations were calculated using the data of four different patient samples. A short description of these independent samples will show the differences and similarities between them.

Samples and Methods

First Sample

During 17 trials with antidepressant drugs 333 patients were examined and the symptomatology assessed with the HAMD and the AMP-System. 101 patients were male and 232 were female; patients were on the average 52.58 years old (s = 12.89 years). We used the expanded 24-item version of the HAMD (National Institute of Mental Health), including the original 17-item version [*Hamilton,* 1960, 1967]. The data were analyzed using the one-dimensional analysis [*Baumann,* 1976], summing up the scores of items 1–17 and 1–24 (one rater).

Second Sample

127 schizophrenic patients were treated with neuroleptic drugs during seven trials. 58 patients were male, 69 female, the age was on the average 41.58 years (s = 12.96 years). We used the German version of the BPRS [*Overall and Gorham,* 1962; *Mombour* et al., 1975]. The data were analyzed with the 4-factor solution [*Overall,* 1974].

Third Sample

In two studies we registered the psychopathological symptoms of 77 patients (one measurement) with the AMP-System and the inpatient multidimensional psychiatric scale (IMPS), German translation by *Flegel, Maeder,* and *Missel* [*Lorr* et al., 1963; *Mombour* et al., 1973], using the 10-factor solution for data analysis. The sample includes 39 male and 38 female schizophrenic patients treated with several neuroleptic drugs. The patients were on the average 37.22 years old (s = 12.37 years).

Fourth Sample

The psychopathological symptoms of 170 hospitalized patients (median = 4 days) were documented (one measurement) with the German version of the comprehensive psychopathological rating scale (CPRS) [*Åsberg* et al., 1978; *Kuny* et al., in preparation] and the AMP-System. The sample includes 73 male and 97 female patients, the average age was 40.10 years (s = 15.10 years). 96 patients suffered from schizophrenia and 74 from depressive syndromes of different etiology.

Based on factor analyses the items of the AMP-System and other rating scales have been used to build up syndrome subscales. Correlations between the syndromes of different rating scales show similarities and dissimilarities which are important for the interpretation of the results obtained with different rating scales. For the following comparisons we used the nine AMP syndromes (primary scales) constructed by *Baumann* [1974] and the two second-order scales constructed by *Woggon and Dittrich* [1979]. Correlations were calculated using the rank correlation coefficient of Spearman (rho).

Table II: Relevant correlations (|rho| ≥ 0.50) between AMP and HAMD, BPRS, CPRS

	AMP			
	primary scales	rho	second-order scales	rho
HAMP				
Score 1–17	hypochondriasis	0.52	manic-depressive syndrome	0.62
Score 1–24	retarded depressive syndrome	0.60	manic-depressive syndrome	0.66
BPRS				
Thinking disturbance	hallucinatory syndrome	0.53	schizophrenic syndrome	0.64
	paranoid syndrome	0.63		
Withdrawal-retardation	apathy	0.57	–	
	catatonic syndrome	0.50		
Hostile-suspiciousness	–		–	
Anxious depression	retarded depressive syndrome	0.60	manic-depressive syndrome	0.53
	hypochondriasis	0.51		
CPRS				
Manic syndrome	apathy	– 0.79	manic-depressive syndrome	0.74
	manic syndrome	0.74		
	retarded depressive syndrome	– 0.59		
	hypochondriasis	– 0.53		
Schizophrenic syndrome	hallucinatory syndrome	0.81	schizophrenic syndrome	0.94
	paranoid syndrome	0.81		
Depressive syndrome	apathy	0.84	manic-depressive syndrome	0.94
	manic syndrome	– 0.50		
	somatic depressive syndrome	0.84		
	retarded depressive syndrome	0.89		
	hypochondriasis	0.83		
Side effects	–		–	

Results

Depending on the size of our patient samples ($n \geq 77$) relative small correlation coefficients ($rho < 0.30$) became significant ($p \leq 0.05$). The practical relevance [*Bredenkamp,* 1972] of such statistically significant correlations is questionable. One can accept correlations as being relevant, if they correspond to an explained proportion of variance of at least 25% [*Cohen,* 1977]. The explained proportion of variance can be obtained by calculating the square of Pearson's product-moment coefficient (r). For the use of the product-moment coefficient the scores should show a normal distribution, which is only the case for the AMP syndromes. Therefore, we used the square of Spearman's rank correlation coefficient

Table III: Relevant correlations (|rho| ≥ 0.50) between AMP and IMPS

IMPS	AMP primary scales	rho	AMP second-order scales	rho
Excitement	apathy	−0.60	manic-depressive syndrome	−0.65
	manic syndrome	0.88		
Hostile belligerence	hostility	0.74	–	
Paranoid projection	hallucinatory syndrome	0.75	schizophrenic syndrome	0.76
	paranoid syndrome	0.73		
Grandiose expansiveness	manic syndrome	0.57	–	
Perceptual distortions	hallucinatory syndrome	0.71	schizophrenic syndrome	0.60
	paranoid syndrome	0.55		
Anxious intropunitiveness	retarded depressive syndrome	0.50	–	
Retardation and apathy	apathy	0.69	manic-depressive syndrome	0.62
	catatonic syndrome	0.63		
	retarded depressive syndrome	0.60		
Disorientation	–		–	
Motor disturbances	paranoid syndrome	0.54	schizophrenic syndrome	0.63
	catatonic syndrome	0.61		
Conceptual disorganisation	manic syndrome	0.60	–	

Table IV: Correlations (rho) between AMP syndromes and HAMD scores (1–17, 1–24) on days 0, 10, and 20 (n=333)

AMP	HAMD first score 1–17			HAMD second score 1–24		
	day 0	day 10	day 20	day 0	day 10	day 20
1 Apathy	0.38	0.64*	0.67*	0.43	0.67*	0.69*
2 Hallucinatory syndrome	0.09	0.31	0.38	0.26	0.41	0.45
3 Hostility	0.20	0.36	0.40	0.25	0.40	0.43
4 Manic syndrome	0.15	0.08	0.09	0.12	0.06	0.09
5 Somatic-depressive syndrome	0.46	0.63*	0.68*	0.36	0.58*	0.64*
6 Paranoid syndrome	0.14	0.49	0.58*	0.31	0.58*	0.66*
7 Catatonic syndrome	0.40	0.66*	0.75*	0.47	0.70*	0.77*
8 Retarded depressive syndrome	0.49	0.71*	0.77*	0.60*	0.77*	0.82*
9 Hypochondriasis	0.52*	0.72*	0.76*	0.48	0.71*	0.77*
S1 Manic-depressive syndrome	0.62*	0.79*	0.83*	0.66*	0.82*	0.84*
S2 Schizophrenic syndrome	0.18	0.42	0.52*	0.33	0.50*	0.59*

rho significant ≥ 0.17.
*rho relevant ≥ 0.50.

Table V. Correlations (rho) between AMP syndromes and BPRS syndromes on days 0, 10, and 20 (n = 127)

AMP	BPRS											
	thinking disturbance			withdrawal retardation			hostile-suspiciousness			anxious depression		
	day 0	day 10	day 20	day 0	day 10	day 20	day 0	day 10	day 20	day 0	day 10	day 20
1 Apathy	0.08	0.16	0.17	0.57*	0.64*	0.72*	0.01	0.10	0.15	0.26	0.35	0.30
2 Hallucinatory syndrome	0.53*	0.71*	0.76*	0.01	0.13	0.13	0.07	0.27	0.48	0.05	0.24	0.37
3 Hostility	0.27	0.42	0.50*	0.07	0.22	0.27	0.45	0.58*	0.66*	0.01	0.23	0.36
4 Manic syndrome	0.38	0.26	0.38	–0.22	–0.16	–0.12	0.07	0.05	0.14	–0.10	–0.05	0.08
5 Somatic-depressive syndrome	0.08	0.23	0.25	0.15	0.17	0.29	0.15	0.20	0.21	0.49	0.42	0.44
6 Paranoid syndrome	0.63*	0.71*	0.78*	0.00	0.13	0.28	0.34	0.41	0.59*	0.23	0.30	0.49
7 Catatonic syndrome	0.27	0.50*	0.55*	0.50*	0.61*	0.60*	0.34	0.37	0.49	0.30	0.44	0.51*
8 Retarded depressive syndrome	0.11	0.32	0.32	0.31	0.48	0.55*	0.11	0.28	0.32	0.60*	0.67*	0.63*
9 Hypochondriasis	0.12	0.30	0.33	0.12	0.49	0.42	0.17	0.27	0.37	0.51*	0.54*	0.61*
S1 Manic-depressive syndrome	–0.07	0.16	0.13	0.36	0.48	0.58*	0.11	0.20	0.24	0.53*	0.53*	0.51*
S2 Schizophrenic syndrome	0.64*	0.78*	0.82*	0.24	0.32	0.37	0.34	0.43	0.60*	0.23	0.37	0.51*

rho significant ≥ 0.17.
* rho relevant ≥ 0.50.

Table VI. AMP and HAMD scores on days 0, 10, and 20 (n = 333; mean ± SD)

	day 0		day 10		day 20	
AMP						
1 Apathy	58.19	± 7.75	53.95	± 8.66	51.27	± 8.77
2 Hallucinatory syndrome	44.12	± 5.75	43.54	± 5.23	43.14	± 4.93
3 Hostility	46.00	± 7.07	44.86	± 7.05	44.02	± 7.05
4 Manic syndrome	44.95	± 4.87	44.41	± 4.72	44.60	± 5.42
5 Somatic-depressive syndrome	58.15	± 5.51	52.17	± 7.31	48.55	± 8.55
6 Paranoid syndrome	45.35	± 6.79	43.31	± 7.03	42.39	± 7.26
7 Catatonic syndrome	53.52	± 7.27	48.93	± 8.18	47.09	± 8.55
8 Retarded depressive syndrome	59.68	± 4.13	54.67	± 7.66	51.34	± 8.99
9 Hypochondriasis	60.44	± 6.89	55.33	± 8.73	52.69	± 9.72
S1 Manic-depressive syndrome	59.33	± 6.16	53.60	± 7.22	50.76	± 7.68
S2 Schizophrenic syndrome	39.73	± 6.43	38.08	± 6.41	37.03	± 6.62
HAMD						
1 score 1–17	25.45	± 7.29	18.68	± 9.01	15.54	± 9.65
2 score 1–24	33.56	± 9.70	24.64	± 12.42	20.57	± 13.42

Table VII: AMP and BPRS scores on days 0, 10, and 20 (n = 127; mean ± SD)

	day 0		day 10		day 20	
AMP						
1 Apathy	50.25	± 8.40	48.60	± 7.66	48.54	± 7.82
2 Hallucinatory syndrome	57.13	± 10.91	51.50	± 9.66	49.56	± 9.09
3 Hostility	56.29	± 7.95	52.11	± 8.44	51.02	± 8.83
4 Manic syndrome	55.28	± 10.34	50.81	± 9.34	49.53	± 8.87
5 Somatic-depressive syndrome	46.00	± 9.06	41.06	± 7.24	39.55	± 6.78
6 Paranoid syndrome	58.93	± 6.77	51.89	± 9.21	49.43	± 10.08
7 Catatonic syndrome	56.83	± 7.75	51.60	± 7.53	50.64	± 8.27
8 Retarded depressive syndrome	50.63	± 7.85	47.54	± 7.95	46.34	± 7.54
9 Hypochondriasis	52.10	± 8.42	48.06	± 7.77	46.86	± 8.02
S1 Manic-depressive syndrome	46.50	± 8.73	44.53	± 6.83	44.28	± 6.07
S2 Schizophrenic syndrome	54.86	± 7.87	48.54	± 7.68	46.65	± 8.05
BPRS						
1 Thinking disturbance	10.92	± 3.91	8.35	± 3.91	7.55	± 3.90
2 Withdrawal-retardation	9.32	± 3.28	7.98	± 2.95	7.92	± 3.34
3 Hostile-suspiciousness	9.32	± 3.68	7.37	± 3.68	7.08	± 3.74
4 Anxious depression	8.84	± 3.47	6.75	± 3.01	6.29	± 3.00

(rho) as a measure for the 'estimated relevance'. Based on this explanation $|rho| \geq 0.50$ is interpreted as being relevant.

The correlations between AMP syndromes (primary and second-order scales) and the syndromes of the HAMD, BPRS, CPRS, IMPS show close similarities (tables II, III). This result shows a good criterion-related validity of the AMP-System.

The highest correlations have been found between AMP syndromes and CPRS syndromes. The reason could be that the AMP-System has a better clinical similarity to the CPRS than to the other three rating scales. Because of the following two methodological reasons this interpretation should be made with caution: (1) The correlation between measured variables is influenced by the errors of measurement, in our case especially by the interrater reliability. The interrater reliability of AMP syndromes was in a recent study [*Maurer* et al., in preparation] much better than in an earlier study [*Baumann and Woggon,* 1979]. (2) Correlations between rating scales can considerably differ in the same patient sample during treatment [*Heimann and Schmocker,* 1974]. We examined this problem in two patient samples. In a group of depressed patients we calculated correlations on days 0, 10, and 20 between AMP syndromes and HAMD scores and in schizophrenic patients between AMP and BPRS syndromes. As shown in tables IV and V most of the syndromes show a higher correlation after 20 days of treatment than prior to the treatment. The change concerns not only syndromes with similar content, e.g., depressive symptoms, but also syndromes of very different content. At first we thought that a changed variance after treatment could be a possible reason. But as shown in tables VI and VII the variance of the different syndromes shows no relevant difference between days 0 and 20. After treatment more symptoms are not present in the patients than prior to the treatment, and according to our experience it is easier to reach an agreement between raters on symptoms which are absent than on present symptoms. Furthermore, one should not forget that the factorical structure of rating scales can change over time [*Woggon* et al., 1980].

Conclusions

The purpose of this paper is to show that to a great extent the AMP-System reflects the clinical picture of severely disturbed psychiatric patients. Furthermore, it is especially suitable to assess drug-induced changes of the symptomatology including unexpected and unwanted effects. Applying the AMP-System, usually no other scales, e.g., measuring side effects, are necessary. Correlated with other rating scales (BPRS, HAMD, IMPS, CPRS) the primary and secondary AMP Scales show a good criterion-related validity. The correlation between these rating scales increases during a treatment. This may be due to a loss of structure of the psychopathological space underlying the factor solution, because the symptoms may become more and more uncharacteristic during improvement.

References

Åsberg, M.; Montgomery, S.A.; Perris, C.; Schalling, D.; Sedvall, C.: A comprehensive psychopathological rating scale. Acta psychiat. scand., suppl. 271; pp. 5–27 (1978).

Baumann, U.: Diagnostische Differenzierungsfähigkeit von Psychopathologie-Skalen. Arch. Psychiat. Nervkrankh. *219:* 89–103 (1974).

Baumann, U.: Methodische Untersuchungen zur Hamilton-Depressions-Skala. Arch. Psychiat. Nervkrankh. *222:* 359–375 (1976).

Baumann, U.; Woggon, B.: Interrater-Reliabilität bei Diagnosen, AMP-Syndromen und AMP-Symptomen. Arch. Psychiat. Nervkrankh. *227:* 3–15 (1979).

Bredenkamp, J.: Der Signifikanztest in der psychologischen Forschung (Akademische Verlagsgesellschaft, Frankfurt/Main 1972).

Carmines, E.G.; Zeller, R.A.: Reliability and validity assessment. Sage University Paper Series on Quantitative Applications in the Social Sciences, 07–017 (Sage Publications, Beverly Hills 1979).

Cohen, J.: Statistical power analysis for the behavioral sciences (Academic Press, New York 1977).

Hamilton, M.: A rating scale for depression. J. Neurol. Neurosurg. Psychiat. *23:* 56–62 (1960).

Hamilton, M.: Development of a rating scale for primary depressive illness. Br. J. soc. clin. Psychol. *6:* 278–296 (1967).

Heimann, H.; Schmocker, A.: Zur Problematik der Beurteilung des Schweregrades psychiatrischer Zustandsbilder. Arzneimittel-Forsch. *24:* 1004–1006 (1974).

Kuny, S.; Maurer, M.; Luckner, N. von; Woggon, B.: Deutschsprachige Version der CPRS (in preparation).

Lorr, M.; Klett, C.J.; McNair, D.M.; Lasky, J.J.: Inpatient multidimensional psychiatric scale (IMPS) (Consulting Psychologists Press, Palo Alto 1963).

Maurer, M.; Kuny, S.; Woggon, B.; Dittrich, A.; Luckner, N. von: Vergleich zwischen AMP-System und CPRS (in preparation).

Mombour, W.; Gammel, G.; Zerssen, D. von; Heyse, M.: Die Objektivierung psychiatrischer Syndrome durch multifaktorielle Analyse des psychopathologischen Befundes. Nervenarzt *44:* 352–358 (1973).

Mombour, W.; Kockott, G.; Fliege, K.: Die Brief Psychiatric Rating Scale (BPRS) von Overall und Gorham bei akuten paranoid-halluzinatorischen Psychosen. Untersuchungen zu einer deutschen Übersetzung der BPRS. Pharmakopsychiatr. Neuro-Psychopharmakol. *8:* 279–228 (1975).

Overall, J. E.: The brief psychiatric rating scale in psychopharmacology research; in Pichot, Psychological measurements in psychopharmacology, pp. 67–78 (Karger, Basel 1974).

Overall, J. E.; Gorham, D. R.: The brief psychiatric rating scale. Psychol. Rep. *10:* 799–812 (1962).

Pecknold, J. C.; Ban, T. A.; Lehmann, H. E.; Climan, M.: Clomacran in the treatment of schizophrenic patients: a comparison of two assessment methods. Int. J. clin. Pharm. Ter. Tox. *11:* 299–303 (1975).

Saarma, J.; Morozov, G.: Experiences with the Russian and Estonian translations of the AMP psychopathology scale in depression and schizophrenia; in Deniker, Radouco-Thomas, Villeneuve, Neuro-psychopharmacology, pp. 1569–1570 (Pergamon Press, Oxford 1978).

Woggon, B.; Dittrich, A.: Konstruktion übergeordneter AMP-Skalen: «manisch-depressives» und «schizophrenes Syndrom». Int. Pharmacopsychiat. *14:* 325–337 (1979).

Woggon, B.; Dittrich, A.; Luckner, N. von; Keller, W.: Unternehmung zur Stabilität der faktoriellen Struktur des AMP-Systems im Behandlungsverlauf. Int. Pharmacopsychiat. *15:* 350–364 (1980).

Prof. Dr. J. Angst, Psychiatrische Universitätsklinik, Forschungsdirektion, Postfach 68, CH-8029 Zürich 8 (Switzerland)

Mod. Probl. Pharmacopsychiat., vol. 20, pp. 185–192 (Karger, Basel 1983)

The AMDP and NCDEU/BLIPS Systems: Similarities and Differences

W. Guy, T.A. Ban

Department of Psychiatry, Vanderbilt University and Tennessee Neuropsychiatric Institute, Nashville, Tenn., USA

Parallel, but independent, development in research is not uncommon. More often than not the times are ripe for several lines of research to come to fruition simultaneously. In the present instance, the explosive growth of psychotropic drugs, the expansion of community-based treatment and the accessibility of computer services made the notion of large, standardized processing systems for psychiatric data a feasible and desirable goal.

In the decade following the introduction of psychotropics, there was an unprecedented burst of research activity which produced new and exciting data. Unfortunately, much of these data were confusing and seemingly contradictory. Attempts at replication often muddied rather than clarified the picture. Differences in terminology, assessments and technique made comparison of findings tenuous if not impossible. It became clear to investigators on both sides of the Atlantic that, to avoid chaos, some common ground for terminology and practice was vital. Thus, it was that analogous methodologies to cope with the problem were developed simultaneously and independently in different areas of the globe. This presentation will concern itself with a brief outline of two such developments – the Association for Methodology and Documentation in Psychiatry (originally AMP, now AMDP and so referred to from here on) and the Early Clinical Drug Evaluation Units (originally ECDEU, now NCDEU and so referred to from here on)/Biometric Laboratory Information-Processing Systems (BLIPS) [5, 7].

Though initiated around the same period of the 1960s, the two systems had different origins. A group of German-speaking psychiatric researchers formed an independent collaborative group – the AMDP. The participants had diverse backgrounds and, consequently, brought many areas of expertise to the task of developing a new and comprehensive system of assessment. The North American group, on the other hand, was somewhat more homogeneous since it consisted of the participants of the NCDEU – a program sponsored by the Psychopharmacology Research Branch of the National Institute of Mental Health (PRB-NIMH). Under this sponsorship, some 20 university-based investigators in the USA and Canada were engaged in conducting clinical drug research on both marketed and investigational psychotropic agents. Each investigator, however, was free to choose his own methods of design and assessment. It became apparent to these researchers as well as to PRB-NIMH that the multiplicity of approaches were generating contradictions and confusions which were most likely a consequence of technique rather than scientific reality. Therefore, a committee chosen from among investigators and from the Biometric Laboratory of George Washington University was formed to develop a methodology to cope with the problem.

Given their concentration in psychopharmacology and in clinical drug research, it is not surprising that the NCDEU group would focus its attention on evaluation in these areas. Of primary concern was the establishment of standard method of assessment and procedure in the conduct of early and late phase II psychotropic drug trials since these types of trials constituted the bulk of their activities. The more heterogeneous AMDP group, however, chose a different path in its attempt to create a common language of research. With a long tradition of descriptive psychopathology, they decided to build a more comprehensive system which would meet more general evaluative needs. With the setting of these goals, the two systems began to develop along different lines and with different strategies.

For the AMDP group, the goal of comprehensiveness required that instrumentation be able to encompass a wide range of symptomatology and psychiatric conditions. A search revealed that no suitable instrument was available and so the group decided to construct new assessment instruments to meet their goals. In constrast, the NCDEU group chose to select from among existing instruments. They decided on a battery of disease-specific instruments, i.e. instruments which consisted of target symptoms of various psychiatric conditions. The initial battery consisted of such well-known instruments as the Brief Psychiatric Rating Scale (BPRS), the Hamilton Depression Scale (HAMD), Clinical Global Impressions (CGI) and the Nurses Observation Scale for Inpatient Evaluation (NOSIE). The selection of these scales reflected the emphasis on behavioral assessment as well as the emphasis on inpatient psychiatric populations which predominated at that time.

Measurement of change under various treatment conditions was the major focus for the NCDEU group and, hence, scales which could be completed rapidly and which had demonstrated sensititivity to change were assembled as the 'standard assessment battery'. Investigators were committed to use this battery in their programmatic work although they were free to employ additional non-standard instruments as well. While also concerned with the measurement of change, the AMDP group had the additional goal of the comprehensive evaluation of psychopathological status – something which was bypassed in the initial NCDEU battery. Both systems developed standard instruments for documenting patient demographic status, adverse reactions, and other ancillary information.

After the selection of an 'NCDEU standard battery', the Biometric Laboratory was given the task of creating a suitable data-processing and analysis system. In doing so, the Biometric Laboratory carried the concept of commonality one step further by developing a standard modular data documentation package for early and late phase II trials. Thus, the Biometric Laboratory Information Processing System (BLIPS) was born. In function, the BLIPS was designed to score, edit, compute derived scores and analyze data from any number of different – though uniformly formatted – assessment instruments. In a similar fashion, modular documentation systems have been developed at several European centers to process and analyze AMDP data. The designs of these systems are remarkably alike insofar as procedures and statistical applications are concerned. The BLIPS, however, is a general processing system which can provide standard documentation for almost any type of evaluative data, while the AMDP-System is restricted to that particular set of assessment data. Interestingly, both systems originally employed op-scan forms, found them unsatisfactory and consequently switched to the key-punch mode.

Neither system has remained unchanged over the years. Extensive modifications, expansions and refinements have taken place in each – although the 'multiple scales' approach of NCDEU and the 'unitary scale' approach of AMDP have been maintained. The goal of NCDEU/BLIPS to provide a general documentation system able to accept any assessment instrument as input has been achieved as has been the AMDP goal of a documented, integrated, and cohesive system of psychopathological find-

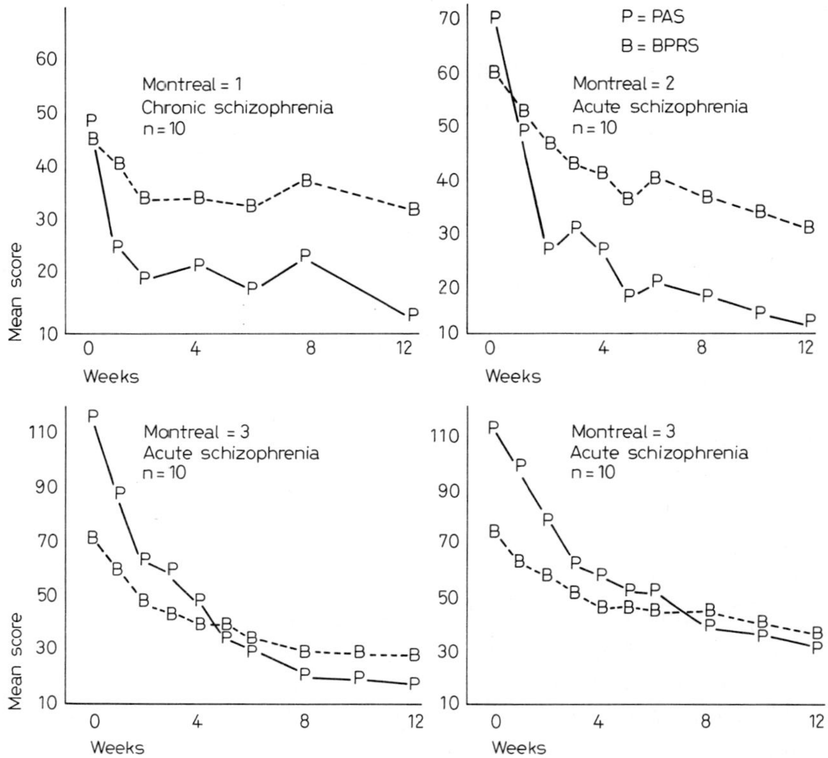

Fig. 1. Comparison of Psychopathological Assessment Scale (PAS) and Brief Psychiatric Rating Scale (BPRS) in four clinical trials involving schizophrenic patients.

ings. These efforts have produced systems which are complementary rather than competitive.

During the early 1970s, one of the original NCDEU participants, the *Lehmann-Ban* group of Montreal, became interested in the AMDP-System and undertook an initial English translation of the Psychopathological Assessment Scale (PAS). When the second edition of the AMDP appeared [9], this group undertook a second English translation of the complete set of instruments including a manual containing an English glossary [4].

Since this group was interested in employing the AMDP in their clinical work along with the NCDEU battery which they had been using for several years, they designed forms for the English AMDP using the NCDEU format. These forms could then be processed by BLIPS. Indeed, AMDP data – primarily the PAS – were subsequently employed and later processed by BLIPS in several of their clinical trials. Data from these trials provide a means of comparing the English AMDP with several of the NCDEU standard scales.

The first set of data involves four 12-week open clinical trials conducted at three clinical units under the direction of the Montreal *Lehmann-Ban* group [8, 10]. These studies involved treatment of schizophrenic patients with investigational neuroleptics using the BPRS and PAS as efficacy measures. Mean total BPRS and PAS total scores across treatment periods for the four trials are presented in figure 1.

In all four trials, statistically significant improvement was reflected by both assessment instruments. Analyses of variance between the two instruments produced no significant differences. Overall correlations between the scales, i.e. across all assessment periods, for each trial were, respectively, 0.86, 0.79,0.81 and 0.77. The more rapid initial drop in PAS scores may be due to the fact that many more areas of psychopathology are assessed on this instrument than on the BPRS; and, as patients improve, only residual pathology – common to both scales – is rated at the latter assessment periods.

The second set of data consists of three double-blind clinical trials comparing an investigational and standard antidepressant. These trials – using a common protocol – were conducted in Montreal, Mexico City and Panama City [1, 2]. The BPRS, PAS and HAMD were employed as efficacy measures. Since the merits of the drugs themselves are not at issue, the samples within the trials have been combined to simplify the presentation. Figure 2 displays mean total scores across assessment periods for the BPRS, PAS and HAMD at each of the research settings.

In the Montreal trial neither statistically significant drug differences nor improvement across time for the sample as a whole were obtained on any of the three instruments. Overall correlations between instruments, however, were positive and significant: HAMD versus PAS = 0.61; BPRS versus PAS = 0.74; HAMD versus BPRS = 0.60.

Statistically significant improvement for the sample as a whole was obtained on all three instruments in the Mexico City trial. In addition, significant drug differences were obtained on the BPRS but not on the PAS and HAMD while the BPRS profile of the combined treatment groups appears to be 'flatter' than those of the PAS and HAMD. Overall correlations between the scales, nevertheless, remain acceptably high: HAMD versus PAS = 0.70; BPRS versus PAS = 0.71; HAMD versus

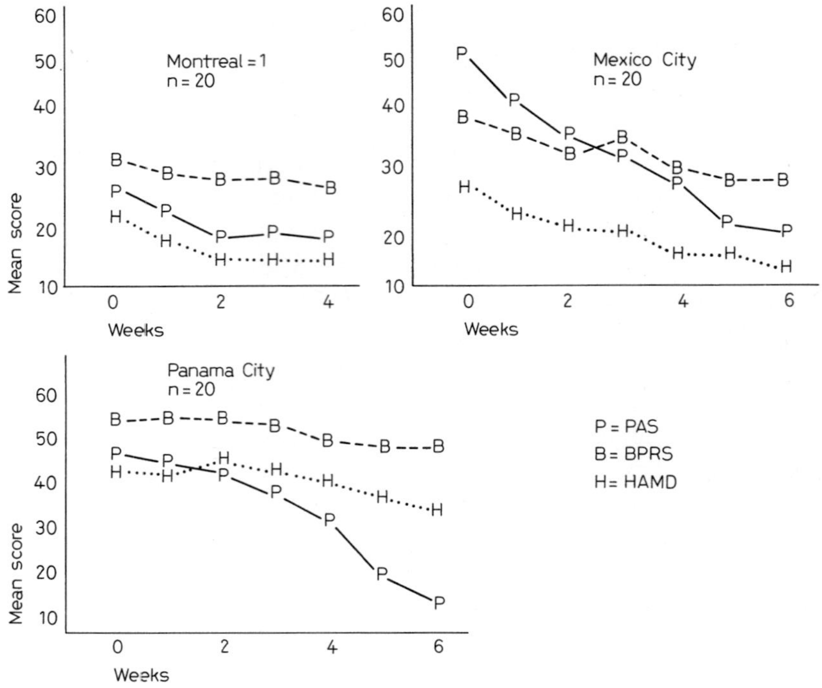

Fig. 2. Comparison of Psychopathological Assessment Scale (PAS), Brief Psychiatric Rating Scale (BPRS) and Hamilton Depression Scale (HAMD) in three clinical trials involving depressed patients.

BPRS = 0.68. The fact that the Mexico City sample was more severely depressed at pretreatment may explain, in part, the disparate outcome with the Montreal trial.

Overall correlations between the scales obtained in the Panama City trial were low in comparison to those obtained in the other two trials: HAMD versus PAS = 0.42; BPRS versus PAS = 0.18; HAMD versus BPRS = 0.50. The rapid drop in total PAS scores – reflecting improvement – which is not mirrored by the HAMD or BPRS, would appear to be the major reason for the low overall correlations. It is not clear from the data, however, why the PAS improvement occurred or why it is not reflected in the ratings of the other two scales.

Despite the Panama City findings, inter-scale correlations across all three trials remain positive and significant: HAMD versus PAS = 0.53; BPRS versus PAS = 0.53; HAMD versus BPRS = 0.60. The profile for

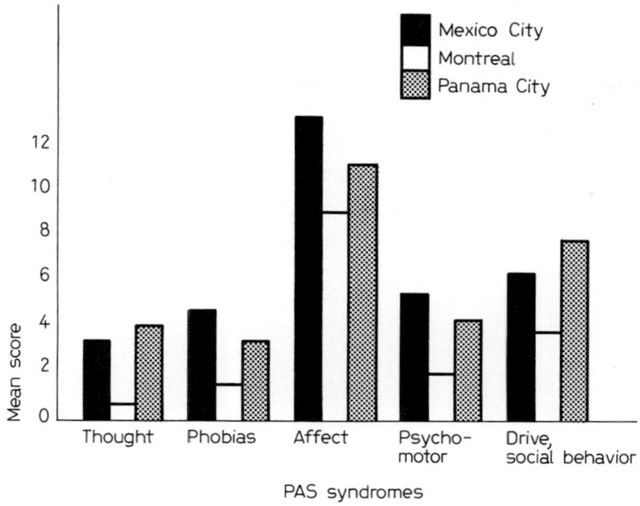

Fig. 3. PAS syndrome profiles for three depressive populations.

each scale is quite similar in each of the three trials. The BPRS shows the least change across time while the PAS shows the most change – perhaps due to its greater psychopathological coverage. An examination of the prominent pretreatment PAS syndromes further reflects the general consistency of ratings (fig. 3).

The profiles for all three centers are remarkably alike – differing only in severity. As would be expected, the syndrome 'Affect' is the one rated with highest pathology with disturbances in Drive and Social Behavior and Psychomotor Retardation being rated somewhat less high. The Mexico City and Panama City populations can be seen to be the more severely ill groups on all syndromes and, particularly, on thought disturbances – suggesting the presence of more psychotic elements than in the Montreal group.Though not a study of reliability in the strict sense, these data demonstrate the compatibility of the major psychopathological instruments of the AMDP and NCDEU/BLIPS systems. Discrepancies may be explained by the differences in scale content; the relative 'looseness' of the translation used and by fact that Spanish – not English – was the mother tongue for several of the raters.

With the increasing concern with nosological problems, there has been renewed interest in psychopathology and its assessment in the USA. The recent publication of the German AMDP-III [3] sparked interest within the Nashville center and, as a result, an English translation of the AMDP-III is now completed [6]. Every effort has been made to ensure the compatibility of the translation with both the original German as well as the French translation – thereby increasing the usefulness of the AMDP-System as a cross-cultural instrument. The availability of the AMDP in the English language will also serve to take more cogent for American psychiatrists a traditional descriptive approach to psychopathology.

References

1 Amin, S.; Ban, T. A.; Lehmann, H. E.: Nomifensin in the treatment of depression: a report on the Canadian part of a transcultural study. Psychopharm. Bull. *14:* 35–37 (1978).

2 Amin, M; Ban, T. A.; Pecknold, J. C.: Nomifensin in the treatment of depression: a standard controlled clinical study. Psychopharm. Bull. *14:* 37–39 (1978).

3 Arbeitsgemeinschaft für Methodik und Dokumentation in der Psychiatrie: Das AMDP-System; 3. Aufl. (Springer, Berlin 1979).

4 Ban, T. A.: The AMDP system in English. Proc. X. CINP, pp. 1575–1579 (Pergamon Press 1978).

5 Guy, W.: ECDEU assessment manual for psychopharmacology. DHEW Publ. No. (ADM) 76-338 (DHEW, Washington 1976).

6 Guy, W.; Ban, T. A.: The AMDP-system (Springer, Heidelberg 1982).

7 Helmchen, H.: State of development of the AMP-system. Drugs exp. clin. Res. *1:* 21–38 (1977).

8 Pecknold, J. C.; Ban, T. A.; Lehmann, H. E.: A standard (trifluoperazine) controlled clinical study with clomacran in newly admitted schizophrenic patients. Psychopharm. Bull. *13:* 14–15 (1977).

9 Scharfetter, C.: Das AMP-System; 2. Aufl. (Springer, Berlin 1972).

10 Torres-Ruiz, A.; Amin, M.; Ban, T. A.; Pecknold, J. C.: Systematic clinical studies with clomacran. II. Standard controlled clinical trials in schizophrenia. Curr. ther. Res. *26:* 127–131 (1979).

Dr. Thomas A. Ban, Vanderbilt University, 1501 Murfreesboro Road, Nashville, TN 37217 (USA)

Mod. Probl. Pharmacopsychiat., vol. 20, pp. 193–203 (Karger, Basel 1983)

AMDP Psychopathology Factors in Chronic Schizophrenia: A Clinical Trial of Two Long-Acting Neuroleptics

Y. D. Lapierre[a], *R. von Frenckell*[b]

[a]Department of Psychiatry and Pharmacology, University of Ottawa, Ottawa, Ont., Canada;
[b]Department of Psychiatry, University of Liège, Belgium

The demonstration of differences in similar treatments applied to a heterogeneous condition such as schizophrenia is limited by the instrumentation utilized in the measurement of the baseline state and of the change brought about by the treatment [*Lapierre,* 1978]. Clinical global impressions probably have the most practical immediate clinical relevance on the broad efficacy of a treatment. However, they generally are not sufficiently sensitive to demonstrate which aspects of the patient's condition are modified in a relevant way by the treatment administered. Behavioral ratings such as the Brief Psychiatric Rating Scale (BPRS) are limited by the broad aspects of syndromal symptomatology which they assess and lack the precision of delineating core symptoms of the illness. The Association for Methodology and Documentation in Psychiatry (AMDP) Psychopathology Rating Scale, by evaluating a vast number of symptoms, focuses specifically on classically well-defined psychopathology [*Guy and Ban,* 1982]. On the other hand, by being exhaustive and specific it has the disadvantage of requiring large numbers of subjects to satisfy the requirements of valid statistical evaluation. To remedy this difficulty, more elaborate statistical methods such as multivariate and principal components analyses may reveal factorization of symptom groups which are statistically valid and clinically relevant.

In this study we compared two phenothiazines, pipotiazine palmitate and fluphenazine decanoate in the treatment of chronic ambulatory schizophrenics over a 1-year period. Previous reports [*Villeneuve* et al., 1972; *Gallant* et al., 1975; *Lapierre* et al., 1979] demonstrated that factor scores of the BPRS were modified in a similar fashion without a clear treatment effect being demonstrated on either treatment. The objective of this study is to determine which of the symptoms interrelate to form factors of psychopathology of schizophrenics prior to treatment and how these may change throughout the period of treatment.

Material and Method

43 chronic schizophrenics of both sexes, aged from 18 to 60 years, were selected as outpatients for this study. The diagnostic categories were compatible with DSM-III Nos. 295.1, 295.2, 295.3, 295.9. An additional inclusion criteria was for the diagnosis to be well-defined for at least 18 months prior to inclusion and the need for continuing neuroleptic medication demonstrated by psychotic relapses having occurred whenever attempts at cessation of the neuroleptic had occurred previously. Clear and well-defined symptoms of active or residual schizophrenic psychosis were required for inclusion. Signed informed consent was obtained for participation in the study. Physical and laboratory examinations of hematological biochemical and electrocardiographic functions were required to be within normal limits. Treatment with pipotiazine palmitate and fluphenazine decanoate was randomized and administered under double-blind conditions. Dosage adjustments were done monthly starting with an initial dose of 12.5 mg and increasing to dosage monthly as required for either control of symptoms or the appearance of side effects. Adjunct medication for extrapyramidal symptoms was benztropine mesylate 2 mg in individually adjusted dosage. Chloral hydrate was the hypnotic permitted when required.

A psychiatric assessment using the first 115-item French version of the AMDP Psychopathology Scale [*Bobon,* 1978] was completed initially and at 3-month intervals by a psychiatrist trained in the AMDP.

The statistical method employed in the analysis of the Psychopathology Rating Scale was principal components factorial analysis. In order to circumvent the problem of disappearance of symptoms with expected improvement during the course of treatment, the initial ratings served as the basis for the factor analysis. The subsequent assessments were projected into this initial structure to compute factor scores on every rating day. Variance analysis for repeated measures on each factor then applied to the intervening variables such as treatment effect and changes during treatment.

Table I. Patient characteristics

	Pipotiazine (14 males, 9 females)		Fluphenazine (9 males, 11 females)	
	X	Range	X	Range
Age, years	31.35	21–49	36.5	19–56
Age on first hospitalization, years	25.7	17–43	28	16–43
Number of hospitalizations	2.6	1–8	2.6	1–8
Dosage (after 52 weeks)				
Males	76.38	12.5 –150.0	65.17	6.25–150.0
Females	78.90	18.75–112.5	49.21	12.5 –125.0

Results

Demographic Characteristics. The patient characteristics are illustrated in table I. The 43 patients, 20 treated with fluphenazine decanoate and 23 with pipotiazine palmitate, were quite similar with no statistically or clinically significant differences between the two groups. The drug administration record of the two neuroleptics required a slightly higher mean dosage for pipotiazine than for fluphenazine and slightly greater doses for males than for females.

Of the 123 items on the AMDP Psychopathology Rating Scale 57 were retained for analysis as they were present in 95% of the assessments throughout the first year. Principal components analysis yielded 10 factors, four of which had factor loadings greater than 0.300 and accounted for 44.78% of total variance. These are listed according to their phenomenological classification including the factor loading score and their contribution to the variance (table II). Thus, a number of items contribute to more than one factor. There is a distinct predominance of cognitive items in factors I and III with mood and emotional disorders items loading negatively in factor III. The negative aspect of mood and emotional symptoms generally load positively to factor I whereas the positive aspects of mood load negatively to this factor. The items dealing with the negative aspects of psychomotor activity load positively in factor I and generally negatively in factors II and III.

Factor I (table III) comprises of the symptoms generally associated with chronic schizophrenia where thought disorders and negative aspects

Table II. Items contributing to main factors

Cluster	Factor			
	I	II	III	IV
Distribution of attention and memory				
Apperception (grasp)	586	–362	312	
Concentration	600		308	
Attention and immediate memory	579			
Distribution of memory	346			
Distribution of thinking				
Inhibited	771			–328
Retarded	700			
Restricted	712		336	
Circumstantial	542		327	
Perseverating	411		513	
Acceleration/flight of ideas		446	314	
Paralogia (tangential)	539		396	
Incoherent/confused	634		378	
Overvalued ideas-compulsions				
Hypochondriasis (not delusion)				421
Delusional ideation/thoughts		665		
Delusional dynamics		624		
Of reference		589		
Of persecution		446	–332	
Ego and personality				
Autism	519		363	
Broadcasting of thoughts				–442
Mood-emotional				
Perplexed	750			
Blunted affect	597	–495		
Affective coldness			–711	
Distribution of vital feelings			–694	
Depressed/sad			–486	483
Hopeless/desperate		431	–573	
Anxious-fearful	430	458		
Elated/euphoric	–534			
Moody-irritable/dysphoric	384	674		
Suspicious/hostile	303	701		
Tense		404		
Inner restlessness			–663	
Full of complaints		592		408
Ecstatic	–574			
Insufficiency – inadequacy	518		–528	
Exaggerated self-confidence	–378			

Table II. Items contributing to main factors (contd.)

Cluster	Factor I	II	III	IV
Guilt feelings		574		
Inadequate affect	549	–571		–322
Emotional lability		605		
Emotional rigidity	529	–409		
Psychomotor				
Lack of initiative and spontaneity	666	–304	–443	
Inhibition of drive	666	–304	–443	
Motor restlessness	352	498		
Logorrhea			388	409
Special features				
Better in evening				–511
Better in morning				383
Drives, etc.				
Reduced contact	747			
Feeling of being ill		558		–436
Lack of feeling of being ill		–394	442	399
Lack of insight in illness	331		405	
Suicidal				453
Aggressive tendencies		490		–392
Difficult to engage in an occupation	481		318	
Eigenvalue	9.87	6.99	5.37	3.65
% Variance	17.31	12.27	9.42	6.40
% Variance relative to factor		29.18	23.18	32.03

of mood expression are positively loaded. The negative loadings of this factor are those generally associated with increased affect.

Factor II (table IV) receives positive loading from the positive pathological features of mood and drive found in schizophrenia. This factor is loaded negatively with the negative mood and drive symptoms associated with schizophrenia.

Factor III (table V) receives positive loading from cognitive and thought disturbances, insight and an equally negative loading from the so-called negative symptoms of mood and drive.

Factor IV (table VI) is positively loaded with depression-related symptoms and negatively loaded with symptoms which are more commonly seen in schizophrenia.

Table III. Factor I

Item	Loading score
Inhibited	771
Perplexed	750
Reduced contact	747
Restricted	712
Retarded	700
Inhibition of drive	666
Lack of initiative and spontaneity	666
Incoherent/confused	634
Concentration	600
Blunted affect	597
Apperception (grasp)	586
Attention and immediate memory	579
Inadequate affect	549
Circumstantial	542
Paralogia (tangential)	539
Emotional rigidity	529
Autism	519
Insufficiency – inadequacy	518
Difficult to engage in an occupation	481
Anxious-fearful	430
Perseverating	411
Moody-irritable/disphoric	384
Motor restlessness	352
Disorders of memory	346
Lack of insight in illness	331
Suspicious/hostile	303
Exaggerated self-confidence	–378
Elated/euphoric	–534
Ecstatic	–574

Table IV. Factor II

Item	Loading score
Suspicious/hostile	701
Moody-irritable/dysphoric	674
Delusional ideation/thoughts	665
Delusional dynamics	624
Emotional lability	605
Full of complaints	592
Of reference	589
Guilt feelings	574
Feeling of being ill	558
Motor restlessness	498
Aggressive tendencies	490
Anxious-fearful	458
Of persecution	446
Acceleration/flight of ideas	446
Hopeless/desperate	431
Tense	404
Inhibition of drive	–304
Lack of initiative and spontaneity	–304
Apperception (grasp)	–362
Lack of feeling of being ill	–394
Emotional rigidity	–409
Blunted affect	–495
Inadequate affect	–571

As the first four factors contributed most significantly to the variance, these were retained for further analysis. The data collected at weeks 12, 24, 36 and 52 of the study were then submitted to variance analysis for repeated measures to detect differences during treatment as well as between treatments.

Factor I changed significantly during the 52 weeks of treatment with both neuroleptics (fig. 1). This change reflected a decrease in severity of

Table V. Factor III

Item	Loading score
Perseverating	513
Lack of feeling of being ill	442
Lack of insight in illness	405
Paralogia (tangential)	396
Logorrhea	388
Incoherent/confused	378
Autism	363
Restricted	336
Circumstantial	327
Difficult to engage in an occupation	318
Acceleration/flight of ideas	314
Apperception (grasp)	312
Concentration	308
Perception	–332
Inhibition of drive	–443
Lack of initiative and spontaneity	–443
Depressed/sad	–486
Insufficiency – inadequacy	–528
Hopeless/desperate	–573
Inner restlessness	–663
Disturbance of vital feelings	–694
Affective coldness	–711

Table VI. Factor IV

Item	Loading score
Depressed/sad	483
Suicidal	453
Hypochondriasis (not delusional)	421
Logorrhea	409
Full of complaints	408
Lack of feeling of being ill	399
Better in morning	383
Inadequate affect	–322
Inhibited	–328
Aggressive tendencies	–392
Feeling of being ill	–436
Broadcasting of thoughts	–442
Better in evening	–511

the symptoms making up the factor. There was no demonstrable difference between the two drugs on this group of symptoms.

Factor II did not change during the 52 weeks of study nor was there any difference between the two injectable neuroleptics (fig. 2).

Factor III fluctuated differently with the two treatments during the period under study. This fluctuation reflected a marked decrease in symptomatology at the final week of assessment for the patients treated with fluphenazine decanoate and a mild increase at week 24 during treatment with pipotiazine palmitate and then a subsequent reduction to pretreatment levels at week 52. Although statistically significant, these variations reflected only minimal change overall and no significant drug differences were demonstrated (fig. 3).

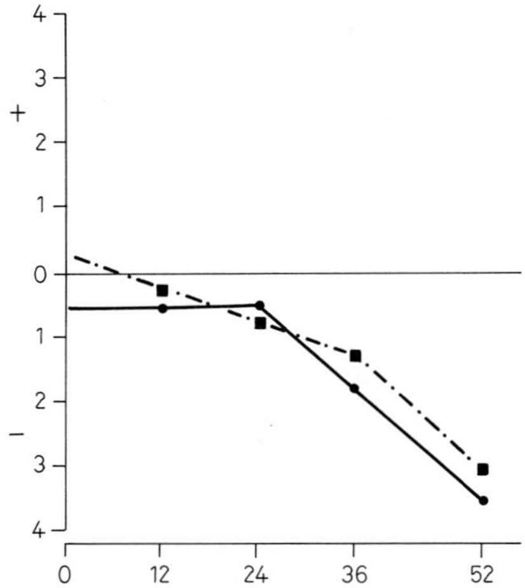

Fig. 1. Factor I. Straight lines = fluphenazine; dotted lines = pipotiazine (F = 23.34, df = 4, p < 0.0001).

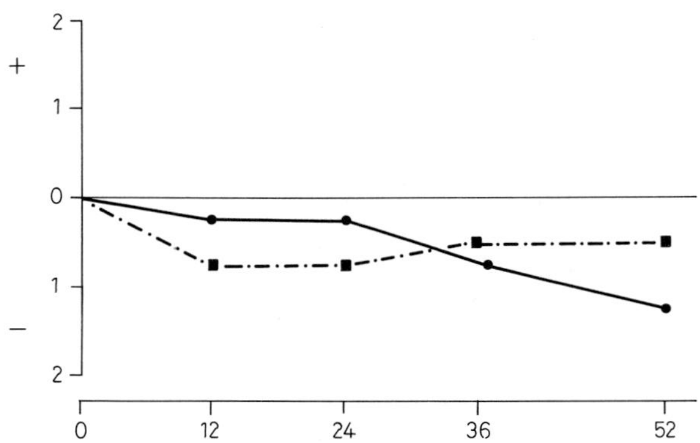

Fig. 2. Factor II. (F = 0.68, df = 4, p = n. s.).

Factor IV also changed significantly during the period under study. The more pronounced change occurred in the patients treated with fluphenazine with only a slight decrease in symptoms observed with pipotiazine treatment. The differences between the two drugs were not significant. It is noted that the patients in the fluphenazine group had higher initial values and ended the study with values similar to those treated with pipotiazine (fig. 4).

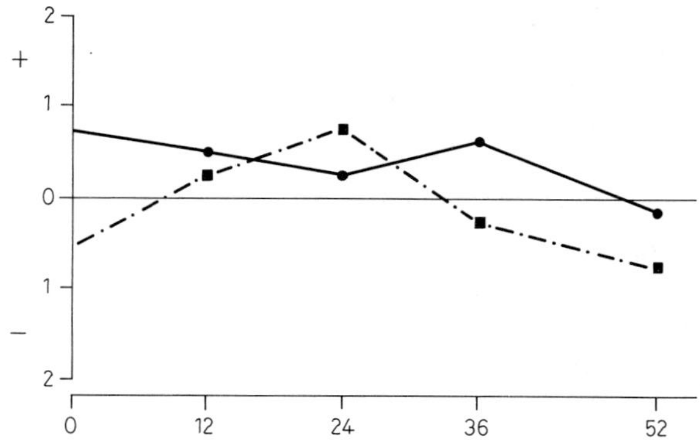

Fig. 3. Factor III (F = 3.67; df = 4; p< 0.008).

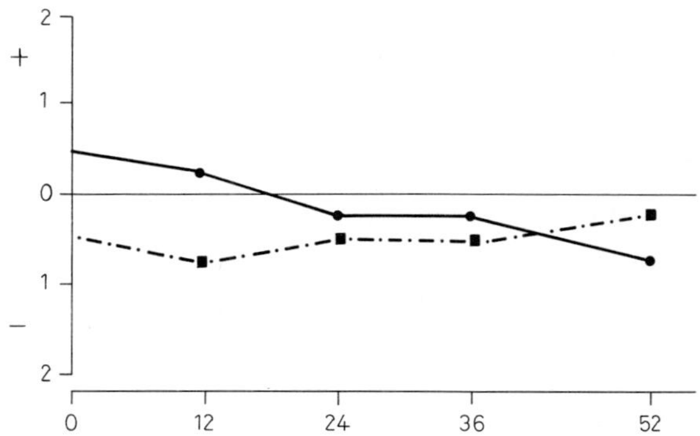

Fig. 4. Factor IV (F = 3.56; df = 4; p< 0.009).

Discussion

This approach in establishing the psychopathological profile of chronic schizophrenics has a dual objective. It is hoped that an exhaustive examination of symptoms using the AMDP-System will better describe the characteristics of a population under study. This then renders possible the establishment of disease and patient profiles which better characterize the population under study. As a further step the validation of the isolated factors by their sensitivity to change with treatment then lends support to the value of the factor. Sensitivity to the demonstration of treatment differences supports their value further. Overriding these caveats is the clinical relevance and logic in the association of the symptoms as a group as conceptual and clinical entities. This becomes the ultimate criterion of value of a mathematical construct.

This approach is not possible unless a rating instrument is sufficiently exhaustive to allow an adequate assessment of the multiple aspects of a syndrome. On the other hand, an overly exhaustive assessment renders statistical validation impossible without a very large number of subjects. In this study the problem was overcome by the use of principal components analysis and subsequent reduction to factors. Those items not relevant statistically were thus logically dropped from analysis. The validation of such factors can be undertaken both within and between studies. In this case the within-study validation was assured by the consistency of the factor throughout the year of observation. Only those symptoms consistently present were maintained for analysis. Whether or not these same factors can be replicated in similar populations remains to be demonstrated. However, in a study by *Bobon* et al. [1983], a similar series of factors were demonstrable in a mixed population. One of these factors closely resembles factor I of our study and may represent the schizophrenics in the sample.

Factor I appears to reflect closely many of the symptoms attributable to process schizophrenia. These are at times referred to as the negative symptoms of schizophrenia which one would generally expect to be most prominent in such a chronic schizophrenic population. Negative symptoms in this case involves thought processes, mood, cognition, interpersonal relationships. These all contribute positively to loading the factor. In the same factor, negative loading is present for symptoms which can be referred to as positive mood. Thus, 'negative symptoms' become associated with absence of 'positive symptoms'. The effect of treatment on this factor is the most pronounced with a marked reduction in the symptoms related to deficiencies in cognition, thinking and drive.

Factor II is positively loaded mainly by positive symptoms related to mood, thought processes and psychomotor activity. The negative loading complements the positive items of factor I. Interestingly these seem to be counterbalanced and do not change significantly with treatment. Possibly, these relatively fixed features are more closely linked to personality features resulting from the illness.

Factor III is formed of symptoms related to cognition for positive and to mood for negative loadings. The more clearly defined cognitive deficiencies are negatively related to symptoms related to mood. These two factors with more equally balanced positive and negative loadings vary little throughout a period of treatment. A similar pattern occurs in factor IV which mainly reflects symptoms of depression, i.e. the neurovegetative aspect of mood disturbance. These latter three factors do not vary to as much as factor I which is more clearly homogeneous in its loading. A further refinement of this statistical method may eventually contribute to precise distinctions.

In spite of these limitations the AMDP Psychopathology Rating Scale provides a comprehensive profile of such a patient population and lends itself well to a clinical drug trial where both the psychopathological profile of the patient and the effect of treatment are of interest. In this case one can state that pipotiazine palmitate and fluphenazine decanoate have a similar pattern of efficacy in the treatment of chronic schizophrenics. Both drugs contribute to improvement of symptoms related to the negative aspects of the syndrome without modifying to as great an extent the stabilized thought disorder and the depressive aspects of the illness.

References

Bobon, D. P. (ed.): Le manuel AMDP (Presses Universitaires, Liège 1978).

Bobon, D.; Mormont, C.; Doumont, A.; Mirel, J.; Bonhomme, P.; Ansseau, M.; Pellet, J.; Pull, C.; De Buck, R.; Gernay, P.; Mormont, I.; Lang, F.; Lejeune, J.; Bronckart, C.; Frenckell, F. von: Analyse factorielle de la révision française de l'échelle AMPD. Résultats d'une étude internationale de 388 cas. Acta psychiat. belg. *82:* 371–389 (1982).

Gallant, G. N.; Mielke, D,; Bishop, G.; Oelsner, P.; Guerrero-Figueroa, R.: Pipothiazine palmitate: An evaluation of a new long-acting intramuscular antipsychotic agent in severely ill schizophrenic patients. Dis. nerv. Syst. *36:* 193–196 (1975).

Guy, W.; Ban, T. A. (eds): The AMDP-system (Springer, Berlin 1982).

Lapierre, Y. D.: Assessment of long-acting neuroleptics: methods and problems. Int. Pharmacopsychiat. *13:* 157–164 (1978).

Lapierre, Y. D.; Berliss, H.; Monpremier, P.; Elie, R.: Methodology and results of a long-term study of long-acting neuroleptics: pipothiazine palmitate and fluphenazine decanoate in biological psychiatry today; in Obiols, Ballus, Gonzales-Monches, Pujol, vol. B, pp. 1087–1094 (Elsevier Biomedical Press North-Holland, Amsterdam 1979).

Villeneuve, A.; Pires, A.; Jus, A.; Lachance, R.; Brolet, A.: A long-term pilot study of pipothiazine palmitate in chronic schizophrenia. Curr. ther. Res. *14:* 696–706 (1972).

Y. D. Lapierre, MD, Department of Psychiatry and Pharmacology, University of Ottawa, Royal Ottawa Hospital, 1145 Carlington Avenue, Ottawa, Ont. K1Z 7K4 (Canada)

Mod. Probl. Pharmacopsychiat., vol. 20, pp. 204–210 (Karger, Basel 1983)

Appendix I:

Applications of the AMP/AMDP-System to Drug Trials[1]

Table I. Some trials with neuroleptic drugs

Neuroleptic	Comparison with	Reference
Baclofen	/	*Beckmann* et al. [1977]
Bromperidol	/	*Bataille* [1978]
	/	*Woggon* et al. [1979]
	Clozapine, Haloperidol	*Woggon* [1978b]
	Perphenazine	*Woggon* [1978b]
		Woggon and Angst [1978]
Cis (Z)-Clopentixol decanoate	/	*Woggon* et al. [1976b]
Clomacran	/	*Galvan* et al. [1976]
Clopimozide	Penfluridol	*Floru and Tegeler* [1978]
Clozapine	/	*Angst* et al. [1971a]
	Bromperidol, Haloperidol	*Woggon* [1978b]
	Haloperidol	*Koukkou* et al. [1979]
Fluphenazine decanoate	Pipotiazine palmitate	*Woggon* et al. [1977a]
		Lapierre and von Frenckell [1983]
	Fluspirilene	*Frei* et al. [1976]
	Fluspirilene, Penfluridol, Perphenazine enanthate, Pipotiazine palmitate	*Angst and Woggon* [1975]
Flupentixol decanoate	Fluphenazine decanoate, Fluspirilene	*Hucker* et al. [1976a]

[1] Adapted from Empirische Studien zur Psychopathologie: Testmanual zum AMDP-System, edited by Arbeitsgemeinschaft für Methodik und Dokumentation in der Psychiatrie, Springer, Berlin, in press.

Table I. Some trials with neuroleptic drugs (contd.)

Neuroleptic	Comparison with	Reference
Fluspirilene	/	*Angst* et al. [1973]
	Fluphenazine decanoate, Flupentixol decanoate	*Hucker* et al. [1976a]
	Fluphenazine decanoate	*Frei* et al. [1976]
	Perphenazine enanthate	*Tegeler and Floru* [1979]
	Fluphenazine decanoate, Penfluridol, Perphenazine enanthate, Pipotiazine palmitate	*Angst and Woggon* [1975]
Halopemide	/	*Bobon* [1983]
Haloperidol	/	*Rüther* et al. [1976]
		Schilkrut et al. [1976]
	Bromperidol, Clozapine	*Woggon* [1978b]
Lenperone	/	*Woggon* et al. [1977b]
Penfluridol	/	*Woggon* [1978a]
	Fluphenazine decanoate, Fluspirilene, Perphenazine enanthate, Pipotiazine palmitate	*Angst and Woggon* [1975]
	Clopimozide	*Floru and Tegeler* [1978]
Perazine	/	*Bente* et al. [1974a]
		Pietzcker et al. [1978]
Perphenazine	Fluspirilene	*Tegeler and Floru* [1979]
	Fluphenazine decanoate, Fluspirilene, Penfluridol, Pipotiazine palmitate	*Angst and Woggon* [1975]
	Perphenazine Oenanthate	*Angst* et al. [1972]
Pipotiazine palmitate	Fluphenazine decanoate	*Woggon* et al. [1977a]
		Lapierre and von Frenckell [1983]
	Fluphenazine decanoate, Fluspirilene Penfluridol, Perphenanzine enanthate	*Angst and Woggon* [1975]
Sulpiride	/	*Bente* et al. [1974b]
		Bobon [1983]
Teflutixol	/	*Bobon* [1983]

/ = No substance in comparison.

Table II. Some trials with antidepressant drugs

Antidepressant	Comparison with	Reference
Amitriptyline	Mianserin	*Vogel* et al. [1976]
	Noxiptyline, Nor-Noxiptyline	*Bente* et al. [1973]
	Amitriptyline retard	*Hucker* et al. [1976b]
Carpipramine	Doxepin	*Athen* et al. [1975] *Woggon and Angst* [1976]
Dibenzepine	Noxiptyline	*Angst* et al. [1971b]
Dexamisole	/[1]	*Bobon* et al. [1974]
Doxepin	Carpipramine	*Athen* et al. [1975] *Woggon and Angst* [1976]
Imipramine	/	*Angst* et al. [1974]
	Lofepramine	*Angst* et al. [1975] *Woggon* et al. [1975]
	Nomifensine	*Angst* et al. [1974] *Woggon and Angst* [1977b]
	Viloxazine	*Floru and Tegeler* [1979]
	L-5-HTP	*Angst* et al. [1977]
	Maprotiline	*Angst* et al. [1972b]
	Ro 8-1998	*Woggon and Angst* [1977a]
	dl-Phenylalanine	*Beckmann* et al. [1979]
Lofepramine	Imipramine	*Angst* et al. [1975] *Woggon* et al. [1975]
L-5-HTP	Imipramine	*Angst* et al. [1977]
Maprotiline	/	*Woggon* et al. [1976a] *Angst and Rothweiler* [1974]
	Imipramine	*Angst* et al. [1972b]
Clomipramine	/[2]	*Bobon* [1978]
Mianserin	/	*Fleischhauer* et al. [1973]
	Amitriptyline	*Vogel* et al. [1976]
Nomifensine	Imipramine	*Angst* et al. [1974] *Woggon and Angst* [1977]
	Nortriptyline	*Pöldinger and Gammel* [1978]
Nortriptyline	Nomifensine	*Pöldinger and Gammel* [1978]
Nor-Noxiptyline	Noxiptyline, Amitriptyline	*Bente* et al. [1973]
	Dibenzepin	*Angst* et al. [1971b]
Opipramol	Phenylpyrrolidinopentan	*Gmür and Angst* [1977]

Table II. Some trials with antidepressant drugs (contd.)

Antidepressant	Comparison with	Reference
Ro 8-1998	Imipramine	*Woggon and Angst* [1977a]
Ro 11-1163	/[2]	*Bobon* [1983]
Viloxazine	Imipramine	*Floru and Tegeler* [1979]

[1] No substance in comparison.
[2] Time-blind evaluation.

References

Angst, J.; Bente, D.; Berner, P.; Heimann, H.; Helmchen, H.; Hippius, H.: Das klinische Wirkungsbild von Clozapin (Untersuchung mit dem AMP-System). Pharmakopsychiatrie *4:* 201–211 (1971a).

Angst, J.; Dittmer, T. L. J.; Heinrich, K.; Hippius, H.; Seibel, I.; Waggon, B.: Klinische Prüfung von Lofepramin im Vergleich zu Imipramin. Int. Pharmacopsychiat. *10:* 65–71 (1975).

Angst, J.; Frei, M.; Beck, M.; Jänicke, U.; Muller, W.; Padrutt, A.; Scharfetter, C.; Vetter, P.; Zulauf, S.: Vergleich von Perphenazin (Trilafon-Tabletten) und Perphenazin-Oenanthat (Trilafon-Depot-Injektion) im Doppelblindversuch. Pharmakopsychiatrie *5:* 169–176 (1972a).

Angst, J.; Frei, M.; Lehmann, M.; Padrutt, A.; Vetter, P.: Comparaison au double insu de la maprotiline (Ludiomil) avec l'imipramine (Tofranil) lors de dépression endogène; in Kielholz, Etats dépressifs: dépistage, évaluations, traitement, pp. 243–250 (Huber, Bern 1972b).

Angst, J.; Frei, M.; Scharfetter, C.: Das Depotneurolepticum Fluspirilen. Pharmakopsychiatrie *6:* 13–28 (1973).

Angst, J.; Jänicke, U.; Peter, J.; Pöldinger, W.: Vergleichende Studie mit den tricyclischen Antidepressiva Noxiptilin und Dibenzepin. Arzneimittel-Forsch. *21:* 635–638 (1971b).

Angst, J.; Koukkou, M.; Bleuler-Herzog, M.; Martens, H.: Ergebnisse eines offenen und eines Doppelblindversuches vom Nomifensin im Vergleich zu Imipramin. Arch. Psychiat. Nervkrankh. *219:* 265–276 (1974).

Angst. J.; Rothweiler, R.: Blood levels and clinical effects of Maprotiline (Ludiomil); in Angst, Classification an prediction of outcome of depression, pp. 237–244 (Schattauer, Stuttgart 1974).

Angs. J.; Woggon, B.: Klinische Prüfung von fünf Depotneuroleptika. Vergleich der Wirkungsprofile von Fluphenazindecanoat, Fluspirilen, Penfluridol, Perphenazinoenanthat und Pipothiazinpalmitat. Arzneimittel-Forsch. *25:* 267–270 (1975).

Angst. J.; Woggon, B.; Schoepf, J.: The treatment of depression with *L*-5-Hydroxytryptophan versus Imipramine. Results of two open and one double-blind study. Arch. Psychiat. Nervkrankh. *224:* 175–186 (1977).

Athen, D.; Bente, D.; Bikadorow, V.; Feder, J.; Müller-Oerlinghausen, B.: Das klinische Wirkungsspektrum mittlerer und hoher Dosen von Carpipramin. Pharmakopsychiatrie *7:* 296–309 (1975).

Bataille, M.: Preliminary note on the antipsychotic efficacy of Bromperidol. Acta psychiat. belg. *78:* 173–179 (1978).

Beckmann, H.; Athen, D.; Olteanu, M.; Zimmer, R.: *dl*-Phenylalanine versus Imipramine: a double-blind controlled study. Acta psychiat. Nervkrankh. *227:* 49–58 (1979).

Beckmann, H.; Frische, M.; Rüther, E.; Zimmer, R.: Baclofen (para-chlorphenyl-GABA) in schizophrenia. Pharmakopsychiatrie *10:* 26–31 (1977).

Bente, D.; Feder, J.; Helmchen, H.; Hippius, H.; Mauruschat, W.: Multidimensionale pharmakopsychiatrische Untersuchungen mit dem Neuroleptikum Perazin. 2. Mitteilung: Verlaufsprofile psychopathologischer und somatischer Merkmale (Untersuchungen mit dem AMP-System). Pharmakopsychiatrie *7:* 8–18 (1974a).

Bente, D.; Feder, J.; Helmchen, H.; Hippius, H.; Rosenberg, L.: Doppelblindprüfung von drei Antidepressiva. 2. Mitteilung: klinischer Vergleich von Noxiptilin, Nor-Noxiptilin und Amitriptylin mit dem AMP-System. Arzneimittel-Forsch. *23:* 247–255 (1973).

Bente, D.; Koeller, D. M.; Koufen, H.; Pietzcker, A.; Schulte, P. W.: Klinisch-statistische Untersuchung des Wirkungsbildes von Sulpirid, einem neuen Psychopharmakon. Arzneimittel-Forsch. *24:* 107–111 (1974b).

Bobon, D.: Time-blind evaluation of psychopathology in drug research. Acta psychiat. belg. *78:* 635–645 (1978).

Bobon, J.; Bobon, D. P.; Bourdouxhe, S.; Pinchard, A.: A pilot open trial of dexamisole (R 12.563) in retarded depression. Preliminary results. J. int. med. Res. *2:* 171–174 (1974).

Bobon, D.: Foreign Adaptations of the AMDP-System. Mod. Probl. Pharmacopsychiat., vol. 20, pp. 19–34 (Karger, Basel 1983).

Fleischhauer, J.; Al-Shaltchi, B.; Brändli, A.: Bericht über eine erste klinische Prüfung von Mianserin (GB 94), einem tetrazyklischen Antidepressivum, im offenen Versuch. Arzneimittel-Forsch. *23:* 1808–1813 (1973).

Floru, L.; Tegeler, J.: Vergleichende Untersuchung der beiden Langzeitneuroleptika Clopimozide und Penfluridol; in Heinrich, Tegeler, Die Praxis der Depotneurolepsie (Tropon, Köln 1978).

Floru, L.; Tegeler, J.: Eine vergleichende Untersuchung der beiden Antidepressiva Viloxazin und Imipramin. Pharmakopsychiatrie *12:* 313–320 (1979).

Frei, M.; Angst, J.; Scharfetter, C.: Vergleich von Fluphenazin Decanoat und Fluspirilen im Doppelblindversuch; in Uchtenhagen, Heimann, Fluphenazin Decanoat-Symposium, Davos, pp. 65–74 (Schwarzeck, München 1976).

Galvan, L.; Torres, A.; Nieto, D.: Clomacran in the treatment of schizophrenic patients. A comparison of two assessment methods. Psychopharmacol. Bull. *12:* 30–31 (1976).

Gmür, M.; Angst. J.: Kombination von Phenylpyrrolidinopentan (Katovit) mit Oxazepam (Adumbran). Ein Wirkungsvergleich im Doppelblindversuch mit Opipramol (Insidon) bei depressiven Syndromen. Int. Pharmakopsychiat. *12:* 100–112 (1977).

Hucker, H.; Woggon, B.; Angst, J.: Schweizerische Studie über die Behandlung mit Depotneuroleptika. II. Präparatspezifische Ergebnisse der Auswertung; in Angst, Burner, Schweizerische Studie über die Behandlung mit Depotneuroleptika, pp. 26–37 (Squibb, Zürich 1976a).

Hucker, H.; Woggon, B.; Angst, J.: Wirkungsvergleich von Amitriptylin (Saroten) und Amitriptylin retard (Saroten retard); in Symposium for Swiss and Dutch Psychiatrists, pp. 51–60 (Lundbeck Laboratories, Kobenhavn 1976b).

Koukkou, M.; Angst, J.; Zimmer, D.: Paroxysmal EEG activity and psychopathology during the treatment with clozapine. Pharmakopsychiatrie *12:* 173–183 (1979).

Lapierre, Y. D.; Frenckell, R. von: AMDP psychopathology factors in chronic Schizophrenia: A clinical trial of two long-acting neuroleptics. Mod. Probl. Pharmacopsychiat., vol. 20, pp. 193–203 (Karger, Basel 1983).

Pietzcker, A.; Müller-Oerlinghausen, B.; Schley, J.; Chaskel, R.; Poppenberg, A.; Urban, R.: Beziehungen zwischen Serumkonzentration und klinischen Befunden bei langfristig mit Perazin behandelten schizophrenen Patienten. Arzneimittel-Forsch. *28:* 1302–1303 (1978).

Pöldinger, W.; Gammel, G.: Differences in effect between nomifensine and nortriptyline. Int. Pharmacopsychiat. *13:* 58–68 (1978).

Rüther, E.; Schilkrut, R.; Ackenheil, M.; Eben, E.; Hippius, H.: Clinical and biochemical parameters during neuroleptic treatment. I. Investigations with haloperidol. Pharmakopsychiatrie *9:* 33–36 (1976).

Schilkrut, R.; Rüther, E.; Ackenheil, M.; Eben, E.; Hippius, H.: Clinical and biochemical parameters during neuroleptic treatment. II Antipsychotic effect of haloperidol in patients with chronic organic brain damage. Pharmakopsychiatrie *9:* 37–42 (1976).

Tegeler, J.; Floru, L.: Eine vergleichende Untersuchung der Depot-Neutoleptika Perphenazin Önanthat und Fluspirilen. Pharmakopsychiat. *12:* 357–365 (1979).

Vogel, H. P.; Bente, D.; Feder, J.; Helmchen, H.; Müller-Oerlinghausen, B.; Bohacek, N.; Mihovilovic, M.; Brändli, A.; Fleischhauer, J.; Walcher, W.: Mianserin versus Amitriptyline. A double-blind trial evaluated by the AMP System. Int. Pharmacopsychiat. *11:* 25–31 (1976).

Woggon, B.: Penfluridol-Ergebnisse einer einjährigen klinischen Prüfung. Int. Pharmacopsychiat. *13:* 1–15 (1978a).

Woggon, B.: Effects and side-effects of bromperidol in comparison with other antipsychotic drugs. Acta psychiat. belg. *78:* 155–172 (1978b).

Woggon, B.; Angst, J.: Das Wirkungsprofil von Carpipramin. Ergebnisse einer offenen Prüfung und einer Doppelblindprüfung gegen Doxepin. Arzneimittel-Forsch. *26:* 2226–2230 (1976).

Woggon, B.; Angst, J.: Open trial and double-blind clinical trial of the antidepressant Ro 8–1998 in comparison with Imipramine. Int. Pharmacopsychiat. *12:* 33–48 (1977a).

Woggon, B.; Angst, J.: Comparison of the efficacy of nomifensine and imipramine; in Alival Symposium Hoechst, pp. 179–187 (Schattauer, Stuttgart 1977b).

Woggon, B.; Angst, J.: Double-blind comparison of Bromperidol and Perphenazine. Int. Pharmacopsychiat. *13:* 165–176 (1978).

Woggon, B.; Angst, J.; Bleuler, M.; Dittmer, T. L. J.; Heinrich, K.; Hippius, H.; Martens, H.; Seibel, I.: Comparison of a new antidepressive Lofepramine with Imipramine in a double-blind multicentre trial. Arch. Psychiat. Nervkrankh. *221:* 157–165 (1975).

Woggon, B.; Angst, J.; Gmür, M.; Hess, K.; Hurwitz, E.; Martens, H.; Rothweiler, R.; Steiner, A.: Klinische Doppelblindstudie mit zwei verschiedenen Dosierungen von Maprotilin (150 und 225 mg pro die). Arch. Psychiat. Nervkrankh. *222:* 13–25 (1976a).

Woggon, B.; Dick, P.; Fleischhauer, J.; Gmür, M.; Gruber, G.; Angst, J.; Heimann, H.: Wirkungsvergleich von Pipothiazinpalmitat und Fluphenazindecanoat. Ergebnisse einer multizentrischen klinischen Doppelblindprüfung. Int. Pharmacopsychiat. *12:* 193–209 (1977a).

Woggon, B.; Fleischhauer, J.; Widmer, A.: Der Einfluss von Diagnose, Klinik und Geschlecht auf die Wirkung von Bromperidol. Int. Pharmacopsychiat. *14:* 213–227 (1979).

Woggon, B.; Franke, A.; Hucker, H.; Rüther, E.; Athen, D.; Angst, J.; Hippius, H.: Antipsychotic effects, side effects and effective dosis of the butyrophenone lenperone (AHR 2277). Int. Pharmacopsychiat. *12:* 113–126 (1977b).

Woggon, B.; Hucker, H.; Angst, J.: Offene klinische Prüfung von Alphaclopenthixoldecanoat (Sordinol-Depot). Symposium for Swiss and Dutch Psychiatrists, pp. 23–29 (Lundbeck Laboratories, København 1976b).

Mod. Probl. Pharmacopsychiat., vol. 20, pp. 211–230 (Karger, Basel 1983)

Appendix II:

Adaptations of the AMDP-System

German

Arbeitsgemeinschaft für Methodik und Dokumentation in der Psychiatrie. Das AMDP-System, 3rd and 4th ed. (Springer, Berlin: Heidelberg 1979 and 1981)

French

Bobon, D.: Le système AMDP, 2nd ed. (Mardaga, Bruxelles 1981)

English

Guy, W.; Ban, T.A.: The AMDP-System (Springer, Berlin, Heidelberg 1982)

Japanese

Manual completed by I. Itoh (in press, Kukusai Isho Shuppan)

Danish

Manual in preparation by P. Bech & M. Kastrup (Hillerød, Denmark)

Greek

Manual in preparation by A. Kokkevi and C. Stefanis (Athens)

Portuguese

Manual in preparation by M. Paes de Sousa (Lisbon)

Spanish

Adaptation: available as microcomputer output (López-Ibor Aliño. El sistema AMDP. Grupo Para El Progreso de la Psiquiatria, Madrid 1980) or as paper-and-pencil form.

Psychiatrie — Anamnese 1

Angaben zur Person

Psych. 1

I-Zahl

0	1	2	3	4		5	6	7	8	9
00	10	20	30	40	Klinik	50	60	70	80	90
	1	2	3	4	Beob.-Periode	5	6	7	8	9
	♂	♀				10	20	30	40	50
	1	2	3	4	Geb.-tag	5	6	7	8	9
	10	20	30						amb.	stat.
	1	2	3	4	Monat	5	6	7	8	9
	10									
	1	2	3	4	Jahr	5	6	7	8	9
00	10	20	30	40		50	60	70	80	90
	1	2	3	4	Geb.-name	5	6	7	8	9
00	10	20	30	40		50	60	70	80	90
	1	2	3	4	Lfd. Befund-Nr. in der Beob.-Periode	5	6	7	8	9
	10	20	30	40		50	60	70	80	90

Datum der Untersuchung

1	2	3	4		5	6	7	8	9
10	20	30		Tag			Okt.	Nov.	Dez.
Jan.	Febr.	März	April	Monat	Mai	Juni	Juli	Aug.	Sept.
1979	80	81	82	Jahr	83	84	85	86	87

Archiv-Nr.

0	1	2	3	4	5	6	7	8	9
0	1	2	3	4	5	6	7	8	9
0	1	2	3	4	5	6	7	8	9
0	1	2	3	4	5	6	7	8	9
0	1	2	3	4	5	6	7	8	9
0	1	2	3	4	5	6	7	8	9

1 Veranlassung der Klinikaufnahme — keine Aussage
freiwillig — unfreiwillig
selbst — Nervenarzt — Vormund/Pfleger
Partner — and. Arzt — Gesundheitsamt
Familie — eig. Poliklinik — and. Behörde
Nachbarn — and. Klinik — anderes

2 Familienstand — keine Aussage — ledig — verh. — verw. — getr. — gesch.

3 Eigene Kinder — nicht zutreffend — keine Aussage — 1 2 3 4 ≥5
Adoptiv/Pflegekinder — nicht zutreffend — keine Aussage — 1 2 3 4 ≥5

4 Biologische Geschwister — nicht zutreffend — keine Aussage — 1 2 3 4 ≥5
Geschwisterähnl. Personen — nicht zutreffend — keine Aussage — 1 2 3 4 ≥5
Zwilling — zutreffend — nicht zutreff. — keine Aussage
Halbgeschw. — zutreffend — nicht zutreff. — keine Aussage
Stellung in der Geschwisterreihe — nicht zutreffend — keine Aussage — 1 2 3 4 5 6 7 8 9 ≥10

5 Alter bei der 1. Heirat — nicht zutreffend — keine Aussage
1 2 3 4 5 6 7 8 9
10 20 30 40 50 60 70 80 90

6 Aufgewachsen (bis 15 J.) — keine Aussage
Großstadt — Kleinstadt — auf d. Land — in wechs. Umgeb.

7 Muttersprache — keine Aussage
deutsch — italienisch — außereurop. Sprache
französisch — and. europ. Spr. — mehrsprachig aufgewachsen

8 Haushalt umfaßt — nicht zutreffend — keine Aussage
Patient — (Ehe)partner — Geschwister
Eltern — Kinder — andere

9 Haushalt wird finanziert durch — nicht zutreffend — keine Aussage
Patient — (Ehe)partner — Geschwister
Eltern — Kinder — andere

10 Anzahl Personen (Haushalt) — nicht zutreffend — keine Aussage
1 2 3 4 5 6 7 8 9 ≥10

11 Anzahl Zimmer (Haushalt) — nicht zutreffend — keine Aussage
1 2 3 4 5 6 7 8 9 ≥10

12 Schulbildung — nicht zutreffend — keine Aussage
Hilfs-/Sonderschule — mit Abschluß — o. Abschl. — in Ausbildung
Volksschule — mit Abschluß — o. Abschl. — in Ausbildung
Mittelschule — mit Abschluß — o. Abschl. — in Ausbildung
Gymnasium — mit Abschluß — o. Abschl. — in Ausbildung

13 Berufsbildung — nicht zutreffend — keine Aussage
Lehre — mit Abschluß — o. Abschl. — in Ausbildung
Fachschule — mit Abschluß — o. Abschl. — in Ausbildung
Hochschule — mit Abschluß — o. Abschl. — in Ausbildung
andere — mit Abschluß — o. Abschl. — in Ausbildung

14 Berufliche Stellung — nicht zutreffend — keine Aussage
Hausfrau — Hausfrau mit Nebentätigkeit
freischaffend/selbständig — selbständiger Unternehmer
ltd. Beamter — Beamter
ltd. Angestellter — Angestellter
qualifiz. Facharbeiter — gewöhnl. Facharbeiter
Arbeiter — anderes

15 Relation zum Beruf — nicht zutreffend — keine Aussage
nicht im erlernten Beruf tätig — ohne Arbeit — arbeitslos gemeldet

16 Ruhestand — nicht zutreffend — keine Aussage
vorzeitig — altersentsprechend — mit Nebentätigkeit

17 Berufssektor — nicht zutreffend — keine Aussage
privater Sektor — öffentlicher Sektor
Land/Forst — Transport/Verkehr
Industrie — Handel
Handwerk — Bank/Versicherung
Dienstleistung (allgem.) — Forschung/Lehre
Militär — anderes

18 Wohnsitz — nicht zutreffend — keine Aussage
Mietwohnung — eig. Haus/Whg. — Gemeinschaftsunterkunft
Untermiete — ohne festen Wsitz — anderes

19 Gesamthaushalts-Nettoeinkommen — nicht zutreffend — keine Aussage
(Mo) ZT: 1 2 3 4 5 6 7 8 9
T: 1 2 3 4 5 6 7 8 9
H: 1 2 3 4 5 6 7 8 9

20 Jetzige Konfession/Weltansch. Bindg. — nicht zutreffend — keine Aussage
protestantisch — jüdisch — and. relig. Bindung — konvertiert
röm.-kathol. — islamisch — nicht-relig. weltansch. Bdg.

21 Intensität Konfession/weltanschaul. Bindung (Patient)
nicht zutreffend — keine Aussage — schwach — mittel — stark

Psychiatrie — Anamnese 2

Angaben zur Person

Psych. 2

	0	1	2	3	4	Klinik	5	6	7	8	9
	00	10	20	30	40		50	60	70	80	90
		1	2	3	4	Beob.-Periode	5	6	7	8	9
	♂	♀					10	20	30	40	50
I-Zahl		1	2	3	4	Geb.-tag	5	6	7	8	9
		10	20	30						amb.	stat.
		1	2	3	4	Monat	5	6	7	8	9
		10									
		1	2	3	4	Jahr	5	6	7	8	9
	00	10	20	30	40		50	60	70	80	90
		1	2	3	4	Geb.-name	5	6	7	8	9
	00	10	20	30	40		50	60	70	80	90
		1	2	3	4	Lfd. Befund-Nr. in der Beob.-Periode	5	6	7	8	9
		10	20	30	40		50	60	70	80	90

Datum der Untersuchung

1	2	3	4		5	6	7	8	9
10	20	30		Tag			Okt.	Nov.	Dez.
Jan.	Febr.	März	April	Monat	Mai	Juni	Juli	Aug.	Sept.
1979	80	81	82	Jahr	83	84	85	86	87

22 Vermutete krankheitsfördernde Einflüsse

nicht zutreffend — keine Aussage

Pat.	Arzt		Pat.	Arzt	
		Liebe			Beruf
		Sexualität			Schule/Studium
		Ehe/Partnerschaft			öffentl. Institution
		Familie			soziale Mobilität
		Finanzen			Vereinsamung
		psych. Beeinträchtigung			körperl. Beeintrg.
		chron. körperl. Leiden			weiß nicht

< 3 Mo — 3 Mo – < 1 Jahr — ≥ 1 Jahr — keine Aussage

23 Veränderungen der Lebenssituation

nicht zutreffend — keine Aussage

0 < 5 J.	5 < 15 J.	15 < 25 J.		25 < 45 J.	45 < 60 J.	> 60 J.	nicht zutreffend	keine Aussage
			Tod Vater					
			Tod Mutter					
1x > 1x	1x > 1x	1x > 1x	Trennung von Eltern ≥ 1 Jahr	1x > 1x	1x > 1x	1x > 1x		
			Trennung (≥1 J.) Scheidung der Eltern					
			Heimaufenthalt (Pat.) ≥ 1 Jahr					
			Heirat (Patient)					
			Trennung (≥1 J.) Scheidung der Ehepartner					
			Tod (Ehe)partner					
			neue Partnerschaft					
			Geburt von Kindern					
			Heirat von Kindern					
			Tod von Kindern					
			Schulausbildung abgebrochen					
			Schulausbildung unterbrochen					
			Berufsausbildung abgebrochen					
			Berufsausbildung unterbrochen					
			Arbeitsplatzwechsel					
			Verlust des Arbeitsplatzes					
			beruflicher Aufstieg					
			beruflicher Abstieg					
			Gefängnisaufenthalt					
			Wohnsitzwechsel					
1x > 1x	1x > 1x	1x > 1x	Suicidversuch	1x > 1x	1x > 1x	1x > 1x		
			Manifestation psychot. Symptomatik					
			Manifestation neurot. Symptomatik					
fragl. sicher	fragl. sicher	fraglich sicher	Alkoholismus	fragl. sicher	fraglich sicher	fragl. sicher		
			Rauschm.-/Medikamentenabhängigkeit					
			chron. körperliches Leiden					
			Endokrine Erkrankung					
			cerebraler Anfall					
			Schädel-Hirn-Trauma					
			and. hirnorganische Erkrankung					

Psychiatrie — Anamnese 3

Angaben zur Person

Psych. 3

0	1	2	3	4	Klinik	5	6	7	8	9
00	10	20	30	40		50	60	70	80	90
	1	2	3	4	Beob.-Periode	5	6	7	8	9
	♂	♀				10	20	30	40	50

I-Zahl

	1	2	3	4	Geb.-tag	5	6	7	8	9
	10	20	30						amb.	stat.
	1	2	3	4	Monat	5	6	7	8	9
	10									
	1	2	3	4	Jahr	5	6	7	8	9
00	10	20	30	40		50	60	70	80	90
	1	2	3	4	Geb.-name	5	6	7	8	9
00	10	20	30	40		50	60	70	80	90
	1	2	3	4	Lfd. Befund-Nr. in der Beob.-Periode	5	6	7	8	9
	10	20	30	40		50	60	70	80	90

Datum der Untersuchung

1	2	3	4	Tag	5	6	7	8	9
10	20	30					Okt.	Nov.	Dez.
Jan.	Febr.	März	April	Monat	Mai	Juni	Juli	Aug.	Sept.
1979	80	81	82	Jahr	83	84	85	86	87
1	2	3	4	akt. Lebens-alter	5	6	7	8	9
10	20	30	40		50	60	70	80	90

24 Jetzige Erkrankung — nicht zutreffend — keine Aussage

Erstmanifestation — zutreffend — nicht zutreffend — keine Aussage

Wahrscheinliche Erstmanifestation im Alter von — keine Aussage

1 2 3 4 5 6 7 8 9
10 20 30 40 50 60 70 80 90

25 Frühere Krankheitsmanifestation

nicht zutreffend — keine Aussage

Verlaufsform — nicht zutreffend — keine Aussage

intermittierend — Vollremission

chronisch — Teilremission

Schwere der Erkrankung seit Erstmanifestation — nicht zutreffend — keine Aussage

zunehmend — gleichbleibend

abnehmend — wechselnd

Wechsel der Symptomatik

zutreffend — nicht zutreffend — keine Aussage

26 Aktuelle Krankheitsmanifestation

keine Aussage

Belastung innerhalb 3 Wochen vor Beginn — somatisch: nicht zutreffend, keine Aussage — psychisch: nicht zutreffend, keine Aussage

Dauer bis zur Aufnahme — keine Aussage

<1 Woche — <1 Monat — <6 Monate — <1 Jahr — >1 Jahr

27 Frühe Störungen — nicht zutreffend — keine Aussage

	zutreffend	nicht zutreffend	keine Aussage
path. Schwangerschafts- od. Geburtsanamnese			
Statomotorische od. Sprachverzögerung			
neurotische Primordialsymptomatik			

28 Psychische Erkrankungen in der Familie

nicht zutreffend — keine Aussage

1. Grades 1 Pers.	>1 Pers.		fernere Verwandte 1 Pers.	>1 Pers.
		Hirnorganische Krankheiten		
		Schizophrenie		
		Affektive Psychosen		
		nicht psychotische Auffälligkeit		
		Art nicht bestimmbar		

29 Suicidversuche b. Angehörigen — nicht zutreffend — keine Aussage

nahe Angeh. — entf. Angeh. — Gesamtzahl: 1 2 3 4 ≥5

30 Suicide bei Angehörigen — nicht zutreffend — keine Aussage

nahe Angeh. — entf. Angeh. — Gesamtzahl: 1 2 3 4 ≥5

31 Suicidversuch des Patienten — nicht zutreffend — keine Aussage

1 2 3 ≥4 sich. SV — letzter SV: <1 Mon. — <½ Jahr — <1 Jahr — <5 Jahre — ≥5 Jahre

32 Abgrenzbare psychiatrische Manifestationen

nicht zutreffend — keine Aussage

mehrere bis 10 — mehrere über 10

1 2 3 4 5 6 7 8 9 10

33 Aufnahmen in psychiatrischen Abteilungen

nicht zutreffend — keine Aussage

mehrere bis 10 — mehrere über 10

1 2 3 4 5 6 7 8 9 10

34 Vorbehandlungsform

nicht zutreffend — keine Aussage

ambulant — stationär — Tag/Nacht-Klinik

allg. med. — allg. psychiat. — psychoanalyt. — Verhalt. ther. — EKT — andere

35 Vorbehandlung mit Psychopharmaka

nicht zutreffend — keine Aussage

Erkrankung	Neuroleptica +	Erfolg	-/?	Antidepressiva +	Erfolg	-/?	Tranquilizer +	Erfolg	-/?
jetzt									
letzte									
frühere									

36 Aufnahmediagnose — Die Zuordnung gelingt — leicht — mittel — schwer

0	1	2	3	4	T	5	6	7	8	9
0	1	2	3	4	H	5	6	7	8	9
0	1	2	3	4	Z	5	6	7	8	9
0	1	2	3	4	E	5	6	7	8	9
ICD	E	N	Y	4	Diagnosen Schlüssel	5	6	7	8	9

37 Entlassungsdiagnose — Die Zuordnung gelingt — leicht — mittel — schwer

0	1	2	3	4	T	5	6	7	8	9
0	1	2	3	4	H	5	6	7	8	9
0	1	2	3	4	Z	5	6	7	8	9
0	1	2	3	4	E	5	6	7	8	9
ICD	E	N	Y	4	Diagnosen Schlüssel	5	6	7	8	9

38 Klinisch-psychiatr. Erfahrung des Untersuchers

unter 1 Jahr — 1 < 3 Jahre — 3 < 5 J. — 5 Jahre u. mehr

Psychiatrie – Psychischer Befund

Angaben zur Person

Psych. 4

Klinik: 0 1 2 3 4 5 6 7 8 9 / 00 10 20 30 40 50 60 70 80 90

Beob.-Periode: 1 2 3 4 5 6 7 8 9 / ♂ ♀ / 10 20 30 40 50

Geb.-Tag: 1 2 3 4 5 6 7 8 9 / 10 20 30 / amb. stat.

Monat: 1 2 3 4 5 6 7 8 9 / 10

I-Zahl

Jahr: 1 2 3 4 5 6 7 8 9 / 00 10 20 30 40 50 60 70 80 90

Geb.-Name: 1 2 3 4 5 6 7 8 9 / 00 10 20 30 40 50 60 70 80 90

lfd. Befund-Nr. in der Beob.-Periode: 1 2 3 4 5 6 7 8 9 / 10 20 30 40 50 60 70 80 90

Datum der Untersuchung: Tag 1 2 3 4 5 6 7 8 9 / 10 20 30 — Monat Jan. Febr. März April Mai Juni Juli Aug. Sept. Okt. Nov. Dez. — Jahr 1979 1980 1981 1982 1983 1984 1985 1986 1987

lfd. Patient.-Nr.: 1 2 3 4 5 6 7 8 9 / 10 20 30 40 50 60 70 80 90

Untersucher: 0 1 2 3 4 5 6 7 8 9 / 00 10 20 30 40 50 60 70 80 90 / 000 100 200 300 400 500 600 700 800 900

Intelligenzstörung (geschätzt): angeb. erworb. n. v. leicht mittel schwer keine Aussage

Beurt.-Zeitraum in Tagen: 0 1 2 3 4 5 6 7 8 9 / 00 10 20 30 40 50 60 70 80 90

Spalten: nicht vorhanden | leicht | mittel ausgeprägt | schwer | keine Aussage

n. v. Bewußtseinsstörungen
1. B.-Verminderung
2. B.-Trübung
3. B.-Einengung
4. B.-Verschiebung

n. v. Orientierungsstörung.
5. zeitlich
6. örtlich
7. situativ
8. über die eigene Person

n. v. Aufmerksamkeits- u. Gedächtnisstörung.
9. Auffassungsstörungen
10. Konzentrationsstörungen
11. Merkfähigkeitsstörungen
12. Gedächtnisstörungen
13. Konfabulationen
14. Paramnesien

n. v. Formale Denkstörung.
15. gehemmt
16. verlangsamt
17. umständlich
18. eingeengt
19. perseverierend
20. Grübeln
21. Gedankendrängen
22. ideenflüchtig
23. Vorbeireden
24. gesperrt/Gedankenabreißen
25. inkohärent/zerfahren
26. Neologismen

n. v. Befürchtungen u. Zwänge
27. Mißtrauen
28. Hypochondrie (n. wahnh.)
29. Phobien
30. Zwangsdenken
31. Zwangsimpulse
32. Zwangshandlungen

n. v. Wahn
33. W.-Stimmung
34. W.-Wahrnehmung
35. W.-Einfall
36. W.-Gedanken
37. systemat. Wahn
38. W.-Dynamik
39. Beziehungswahn
40. Beeinträcht.-Verfolg.-Wahn
41. Eifersuchtswahn
42. Schuldwahn
43. Verarmungswahn
44. hypochondr. Wahn
45. Größenwahn
46. andere Wahninhalte

n. v. Sinnestäuschungen
47. Illusionen
48. Stimmenhören
49. andere akust. Halluzinationen
50. optische Halluzinationen
51. Körperhalluzinationen
52. Geruchs-/Geschmackshallu.

n. v. Ich-Störungen
53. Derealisation
54. Depersonalisation
55. Gedankenausbreitung
56. Gedankenentzug
57. Gedankeneingebung
58. and. Fremdbeeinfluss.-erl.

n. v. Störungen der Affektivität
59. ratlos
60. Gefühl d. Gefühllosigkeit
61. affektarm
62. Störung der Vitalgefühle
63. deprimiert
64. hoffnungslos
65. ängstlich
66. euphorisch
67. dysphorisch
68. gereizt
69. innerlich unruhig
70. klagsam/jammerig
71. Insuffizienzgefühle
72. gest. Selbstwertgefühle
73. Schuldgefühle
74. Verarmungsgefühle
75. ambivalent
76. Parathymie
77. affektlabil
78. affektinkontinent
79. affektstarr

n. v. Antriebs- und psychomot. Störungen
80. antriebsarm
81. antriebsgehemmt
82. antriebsgesteigert
83. motorisch unruhig
84. Parakinesen
85. maniriert/bizarr
86. theatralisch
87. mutistisch
88. logorrhoisch

n. v. Circadiane Besonderheiten
89. morgens schlechter
90. abends schlechter
91. abends besser

n. v. Andere Störungen
92. sozialer Rückzug
93. soziale Umtriebigkeit
94. Aggressivität
95. Suizidalität
96. Selbstbeschädigung
97. Mangel an Krankh.gefühl
98. Mangel an Krankh.eins.
99. Ablehnung d. Behandlung
100. pflegebedürftig

R1 R2 R3 R4 R5 R6 R7 R8 R9 R10 R11 R12 R13 R14 R15

Befundunsicherheit

Psychiatrie – Somatischer Befund

Angaben zur Person

Psych. 5

Klinik	0	1	2	3	4	5	6	7	8	9
	00	10	20	30	40	50	60	70	80	90
Beob. Periode		1	2	3	4	5	6	7	8	9
	♂	♀				10	20	30	40	50
Geb. Tag		1	2	3	4	5	6	7	8	9
		10	20	30					amb.	stat.
Monat		1	2	3	4	5	6	7	8	9
		10								
Jahr		1	2	3	4	5	6	7	8	9
	00	10	20	30	40	50	60	70	80	90
Geb.-Name		1	2	3	4	5	6	7	8	9
	00	10	20	30	40	50	60	70	80	90
lfd. Befund-Nr. in der Beob.-Periode		1	2	3	4	5	6	7	8	9
		10	20	30	40	50	60	70	80	90

I-Zahl

Datum der Untersuchung – Tag		1	2	3	4	5	6	7	8	9
		10	20	30				Okt.	Nov.	Dez.
Monat		Jan.	Febr.	März	April	Mai	Juni	Juli	Aug.	Sept.
Jahr		1979	1980	1981	1982	1983	1984	1985	1986	1987
Prüf-Behandlungstag H	0	1	2	3	4	5	6	7	8	9
Z	0	1	2	3	4	5	6	7	8	9
E	0	1	2	3	4	5	6	7	8	9
lfd. Patient.-Nr.		1	2	3	4	5	6	7	8	9
		10	20	30	40	50	60	70	80	90
Reserve ZT	0	1	2	3	4	5	6	7	8	9
T	0	1	2	3	4	5	6	7	8	9
H	0	1	2	3	4	5	6	7	8	9
Z	0	1	2	3	4	5	6	7	8	9
E	0	1	2	3	4	5	6	7	8	9
Beurteil.-zeitraum in Tagen	0	1	2	3	4	5	6	7	8	9
	00	10	20	30	40	50	60	70	80	90

		nicht vorhanden	leicht	mittel ausgepr.	schwer	keine Aussage
	Schlaf- u. Vigilanz-Störungen (n.v.)					
101.	Einschlafstörungen					
102.	Durchschlafstörungen					
103.	Verkürzung d. Schlafdauer					
104.	Früherwachen					
105.	Müdigkeit					
	Appetenzstörungen (n.v.)					
106.	Appetit vermindert					
107.	Appetit vermehrt					
108.	Durst vermehrt					
109.	Sexualität vermindert					
	Gastro-intestinale Störungen (n.v.)					
110.	Hypersalivation					
111.	Mundtrockenheit					
112.	Übelkeit					
113.	Erbrechen					
114.	Magenbeschwerden					
115.	Obstipation					
116.	Diarrhoe					
	Kardio-respiratorische Störungen (n.v.)					
117.	Atembeschwerden					
118.	Schwindel					
119.	Herzklopfen					
120.	Herzdruck					
	Andere vegetative Störungen (n.v.)					
121.	Akkommodationsstörungen					
122.	Schwitzen vermehrt					
123.	Seborrhoe					
124.	Miktionsstörungen					
125.	Menstruationsstörungen					
	Weitere Störungen (n.v.)					
126.	Kopfdruck					
127.	Rückenbeschwerden					
128.	Schweregefühl i.d. Beinen					
129.	Hitzegefühl					
130.	Frösteln					
131.	Konversionssymptome					
	Neurologische Störungen (n.v.)					
132.	Rigor					
133.	Muskeltonus erniedrigt					
134.	Tremor					
135.	Dyskinesien					
136.	Hypokinesien					
137.	Akathisie					
138.	Ataxie					
139.	Nystagmus					
140.	Parästhesien					
	R1					
	R2					
	R3					
	R4					
	R5					
	R6					
	R7					

Seitendifferenzen NEIN JA

Cerebrale Krampfanfälle NEIN JA

Messwerte

ETABLISSEMENT :

EXAMINATEUR :

ECHELLE PSYCHOPATHOLOGIQUE AMDP - 4

Nom + prénom MALADE	N° de dossier du malade
....	N° du malade dans l'étude
SEXE :	Sexe (M = 1 ; F = 2)
DATE DE NAISSANCE :	Age
DIAGNOSTIC :	Diagnostic CIM-9
....	
DATE DE L'EXAMEN :	Date de l'examen
PERIODE CODEE (jours) :	Nombre de jours évalués

DATE DE LA COTATION VIDEO éventuelle :

MODERATEUR :

Cotation : 0 absent – 1 léger – 2 moyen – 3 fort – 4 très fort – (5) sans avis

Troubles de la conscience (aucun □)
1 Baisse de vigilance
2 Dissolution de conscience
3 Rétrécissement de conscience
4 Expansion de conscience

Troubles de l'orientation (aucun □)
5 T.O. dans le temps
6 T.O. dans l'espace
7 T.O. quant à la situation
8 T.O. quant à sa personne

Troubles de l'attention et de la mémoire (aucun □)
9 Troubles de l'aperception
10 Troubles de la concentration
11 Troubles de la mémorisation
12 Troubles de l'évocation
13 Confabulation
14 Paramnésies / Hypermnésies

Troubles formels de pensée (aucun □)
15 Pensée inhibée
16 Pensée ralentie
17 Pensée circonstanciée
18 Pensée appauvrie
19 Persévération verbale
20 Ruminations
21 Pensée automatique
22 Fuite des idées
23 Réponses à côté
24 Pensée barrée
25 Pensée incohérente
26 Néologismes

Craintes et obsessions (aucun □)
27 Méfiance
28 Hypocondrie non délirante
29 Phobies
30 Obsessions
31 Obsessions-impulsions
32 Compulsions

Délire (aucun □)
33 Pressentiment délirant
34 Perception délirante
35 Intuition délirante
36 Idées délirantes non systématis.
37 Systématisation du délire
38 Dynamisme du délire
39 Idées délirantes de référence
40 I.D. de préjudice/persécution
41 I.D. de jalousie
42 I.D. de culpabilité
43 I.D. de ruine
44 I.D. hypocondriaques
45 I.D. de grandeur
46 I.D. fantastiques

Troubles des perceptions (aucun □)
47 Illusions
48 Hallucinations acousticoverbales
49 Autres hallucinations auditives
50 Hallucinations visuelles
51 Hallucinations cénesthésiques
52 Hallucin. olfactives/gustatives

Troubles du moi (aucun □)
53 Etrangeté
54 Dépersonnalisation
55 Devinement de la pensée
56 Vol de la pensée
57 Pensées imposées
58 Autres sentiments d'influence

Troubles affectifs (aucun □)
59 Perplexité
60 Anesthésie affective (éprouvée)
61 Anesthésie affective (observée)
62 Troubles de l'éprouvé vital
63 Tristesse
64 Perte d'espoir
65 Anxiété psychique éprouvée
66 Euphorie
67 Dysphorie
68 Irritabilité
69 Agitation intérieure
70 Propension à se plaindre
71 Sentiment d'insuffisance
72 Surestimation de soi
73 Sentiment de culpabilité
74 Sentiment de ruine
75 Ambivalence affective
76 Discordance affective
77 Labilité affective
78 Hyperémotivité
79 Monotonie affective

Troubles de l'énergie vitale et de la psychomotricité (aucun □)
80 Diminution de l'énergie
81 Inhibition de l'énergie
82 Augmentation de l'énergie
83 Agitation motrice

84 Parakinésies
85 Maniérisme/bizarreries
86 Théâtralisme
87 Laconisme
88 Logorrhée

Particularités nycthémérales (aucun □)
89 Aggravation matinale
90 Aggravation vespérale
91 Amélioration vespérale

Autres troubles psych. (aucun □)
92 Sociabilité diminuée
93 Sociabilité excessive
94 Agressivité
95 Tendances suicidaires
96 Automutilations
97 Absence sent. d'être malade
98 Non-conscience de la maladie
99 Refus du traitement
100 Besoin de soins

Items de réserve psych. (aucun □)
P1 Fabulation non délirante
P2 Perte du désir de vivre
P3 Asthénie
P4 Pensée accélérée
P5 Tension
P6 Tendance à dramatiser
P7 Anticipation anxieuse
P8 Anxiété en situation sociale
P9 Anxiété observée
P10 Désir sexuel diminué
P11 Désir sexuel exacerbé
P12 Insatisfaction sexuelle
P13 Déviation sexuelle
P14 Pseudo-hallucin. (Hallucinose)
P15 Invalidation sociale

Difficulté de l'évaluation □ □ □ □ □

absent 0 – léger 1 – moyen 2 – fort 3 – très fort 4 – sans avis (5)

ETABLISSEMENT :

EXAMINATEUR :

ECHELLE SOMATIQUE AMDP - 5

Nom + prénom MALADE . . . .

. . . .

SEXE : . . . .

DATE DE NAISSANCE : . . . .

DIAGNOSTIC : . . . .

. . . .

DATE DE L'EXAMEN : . . . .

PERIODE CODEE (jours) : . . . .

└┴┴┴┴┴┴┘	N° de dossier du malade
└┴┴┴┘	N° du malade dans l'étude
└┘	Sexe (M = 1 ; F = 2)
└┴┘	Age
└┴┴┴┘	Diagnostic CIM-9
└┴┴┴┴┴┴┘	Date de l'examen
└┴┘	Nombre de jours évalués

	0 absent	1 léger	2 moyen	3 fort	4 très fort	(5) sans avis
Troubles de la vigilance (aucun □)						
101 Difficultés d'endorm.	□	□	□	□	□	□
102 Réveils nocturnes	□	□	□	□	□	□
103 Dimin. durée sommeil	□	□	□	□	□	□
104 Réveil matinal	□	□	□	□	□	□
105 Somnolence diurne	□	□	□	□	□	□
Troubles de l'appétence (aucun □)						
106 Appétit diminué	□	□	□	□	□	□
107 Appétit augmenté	□	□	□	□	□	□
108 Soif augmentée	□	□	□	□	□	□
109 Impuissance / Frigidité	□	□	□	□	□	□
Troubles gastro-intestinaux (aucun □)						
110 Hypersalivation	□	□	□	□	□	□
111 Sécheresse de bouche	□	□	□	□	□	□
112 Nausées	□	□	□	□	□	□
113 Vomissements	□	□	□	□	□	□
114 Plaintes gastriques	□	□	□	□	□	□
115 Constipation	□	□	□	□	□	□
116 Diarrhée	□	□	□	□	□	□
Troubles cardio-respiratoires (aucun □)						
117 Difficulté à respirer	□	□	□	□	□	□
118 Vertiges	□	□	□	□	□	□
119 Palpitations	□	□	□	□	□	□
120 Précordialgies	□	□	□	□	□	□
Autres troubles végétatifs (aucun □)						
121 Troubles d'accomodation	□	□	□	□	□	□
122 Sudations profuses	□	□	□	□	□	□
123 Séborrhée	□	□	□	□	□	□
124 Miction difficile	□	□	□	□	□	□
125 Troubles menstruels	□	□	□	□	□	□
Autres troubles somatiques (aucun □)						
126 Plaintes céphaliques	□	□	□	□	□	□
127 Lombalgies / Dorsalgies	□	□	□	□	□	□
128 Lourdeur de jambes	□	□	□	□	□	□
129 Sensation de chaleur	□	□	□	□	□	□
130 Frilosité	□	□	□	□	□	□
131 Symptômes de conversion	□	□	□	□	□	□
Troubles neurologiques (aucun □)						
132 Hypertonie extrapyram.	□	□	□	□	□	□
133 Hypotonie	□	□	□	□	□	□
134 Tremor	□	□	□	□	□	□
135 Crises dyskin. aiguës	□	□	□	□	□	□
136 Hypokinésie / Hypomimie	□	□	□	□	□	□
137 Akathisie / Tasikinésie	□	□	□	□	□	□
138 Ataxie	□	□	□	□	□	□
139 Nystagmus	□	□	□	□	□	□
140 Paresthésies	□	□	□	□	□	□
Items de réserve soma. (aucun □)						
S1 Anxiété somatique	□	□	□	□	□	□
S2 Rêves / Cauchemars	□	□	□	□	□	□
S3 Ejaculation retardée	□	□	□	□	□	□
S4 Réactions allergiques	□	□	□	□	□	□
S5 Tics / Bégaiement	□	□	□	□	□	□
S6 Dyskinésies tardives	□	□	□	□	□	□
S7 Oedèmes malléolaires	□	□	□	□	□	□

Asym. neurol. Non □ Oui □

Crises Epi. Non □ Oui □

MESURES :

Poids (Kg)	└─┴─┴─┘	(ex. : 036)
Température (°C)	└─┴─┴─┘	(ex. : 374)
Pouls (/mn)	└─┴─┴─┘	(ex. : 072)
PA couché, max. (mm Hg)	└─┴─┴─┘	(ex. : 135)
PA couché, min. (mm Hg)	└─┴─┴─┘	(ex. : 080)
PA debout, max. (mm Hg)	└─┴─┴─┘	
PA debout, min. (mm Hg)	└─┴─┴─┘	

ENTRETIEN SOMATIQUE STANDARDISE (F)

Comment vous sentez-vous physiquement (ces derniers jours) ?
Bien dormi ? (101 - 104) Pas rêvé ? (S2) Pas somnolent pendant la journée ? (105)
Bon appétit ? (106, 107) Buvez pas plus que d'habitude ? (108, 111)
Pas de troubles digestifs ? Allez à selles et urinez normalement ? (112-116, 124)
Pas de difficultés à respirer ? (117) Pas de vertiges ? (118) Pas la vue brouillée ? (121)
Pas le coeur qui bat trop fort ou trop vite ? (119, 120)
Pas les jambes lourdes, les chevilles qui gonflent ? (128, S7)
Pas anormalement frileux ou trop chaud ? (129, 130) Transpirez pas plus que d'habitude ? (122) Pas de boutons ou autre maladie de la peau ? (123, S4)
Mal nulle part ? (114, 126, 127, S1) Pas de picotements ? (140)
Selon les cas : réglée normalement ? (125) Pas remarqué l'apparition d'une frigidité / difficulté d'éjaculation ? (109)
Autre symptôme physique à signaler ?

REMARQUES INDIVIDUELLES :

HOSPITAL/CLINIC
RATER:

PSYCHOPATHOLOGICAL SYMPTOMS
AMDP - 4

PATIENT INITIALS ___ ___ (1st Last) PT. NO.________

SEX: M___ F___

BIRTH DATE:________________

RACE: W__ B__ I__ O__ OTH________

DATE OF EXAMINATION: ___/___/___ (M D Y)

└┴┴┴┴┴┘	Patient Number
└┴┴┴┘	Study Number
└┘	Sex (M = 1; F = 2)
└┴┘	Age
└┘	Race (W=1, B=2, I=3, O=4, Oth=5)
└┴┴┘	Date of Examination
└┴┘	Period

INTELLECTUAL DEFICIT

1	2	3	4	5	(9)
AB	MI	MO	SV	EX	NA

Inherited _____ Acquired _____

	0 AB	1 MI	2 MO	3 SV	4 EX	(9) NA
DISORDERS OF CONSCIOUSNESS (None □)						
1 Lowered	□	□	□	□	□	□
2 Clouded	□	□	□	□	□	□
3 Narrowed	□	□	□	□	□	□
4 Expanded	□	□	□	□	□	□
DISORDERS OF ORIENTATION (None □)						
5 Time	□	□	□	□	□	□
6 Place	□	□	□	□	□	□
7 Situation	□	□	□	□	□	□
8 Self	□	□	□	□	□	□
DISTURBANCES OF ATTENTION & MEMORY (None □)						
9 Apperception	□	□	□	□	□	□
10 Concentration	□	□	□	□	□	□
11 Memorization	□	□	□	□	□	□
12 Retention	□	□	□	□	□	□
13 Confabulation	□	□	□	□	□	□
14 Paramesias	□	□	□	□	□	□
FORMAL DISORDERS OF THOUGHT (None □)						
15 Inhibited thinking	□	□	□	□	□	□
16 Retarded thinking	□	□	□	□	□	□
17 Circumstant. think.	□	□	□	□	□	□
18 Restricted thinking	□	□	□	□	□	□
19 Perseveration	□	□	□	□	□	□
20 Rumination	□	□	□	□	□	□
21 Pressured thinking	□	□	□	□	□	□
22 Flight of ideas	□	□	□	□	□	□
23 Tangential thinking	□	□	□	□	□	□
24 Blocking	□	□	□	□	□	□
25 Incoherence	□	□	□	□	□	□
26 Neologisms	□	□	□	□	□	□
PHOBIAS AND COMPULSIONS (None □)						
27 Suspiciousness	□	□	□	□	□	□
28 Hypochondriasis	□	□	□	□	□	□
29 Phobias	□	□	□	□	□	□
30 Obsess. thought	□	□	□	□	□	□
31 Comp. impulse	□	□	□	□	□	□
32 Comp. action	□	□	□	□	□	□
DELUSIONS (None □)						
33 Del. mood	□	□	□	□	□	□
34 Del. perception	□	□	□	□	□	□
35 Sudden del. idea	□	□	□	□	□	□
36 Delusional ideas	□	□	□	□	□	□
37 Systematic del.	□	□	□	□	□	□
38 Del. dynamics	□	□	□	□	□	□
39 Del. reference	□	□	□	□	□	□
40 Del. persecution	□	□	□	□	□	□
41 Del. jealousy	□	□	□	□	□	□
42 Del. guilt	□	□	□	□	□	□
43 Del. impoverishment	□	□	□	□	□	□
44 Hypochon. del.	□	□	□	□	□	□
45 Del. grandeur	□	□	□	□	□	□
46 Oth. delusions	□	□	□	□	□	□
DISORDERS OF PERCEPTION (None □)						
47 Illusions	□	□	□	□	□	□
48 Verbal halluc.	□	□	□	□	□	□
49 Oth. aud. halluc.	□	□	□	□	□	□
50 Visual halluc.	□	□	□	□	□	□
51 Bodily halluc.	□	□	□	□	□	□
52 Olf/gust halluc.	□	□	□	□	□	□
DISORDERS OF EGO (None □)						
53 Derealization	□	□	□	□	□	□
54 Depersonalization	□	□	□	□	□	□
55 Broadcasting	□	□	□	□	□	□
56 Withdrawal	□	□	□	□	□	□
57 Insertion	□	□	□	□	□	□
58 Other symptoms	□	□	□	□	□	□
DISTURBANCES OF AFFECT (None □)						
59 Perplexity	□	□	□	□	□	□
60 Loss of feeling	□	□	□	□	□	□
61 Blunted affect	□	□	□	□	□	□
62 Loss vitality	□	□	□	□	□	□
63 Depressed mood	□	□	□	□	□	□
64 Hopelessness	□	□	□	□	□	□
65 Anxiety	□	□	□	□	□	□
66 Euphoria	□	□	□	□	□	□
67 Dysphoria	□	□	□	□	□	□
68 Irritability	□	□	□	□	□	□
69 Inner restless.	□	□	□	□	□	□
70 Complaintive	□	□	□	□	□	□
71 Inadequacy	□	□	□	□	□	□
72 Exag. self-esteem	□	□	□	□	□	□
73 Feeling of guilt	□	□	□	□	□	□
74 Feel. impoverish.	□	□	□	□	□	□
75 Ambivalence	□	□	□	□	□	□
76 Parathymia	□	□	□	□	□	□
77 Affect. lability	□	□	□	□	□	□
78 Affect. incon.	□	□	□	□	□	□
79 Affect. rigidity	□	□	□	□	□	□
DISORDERS OF DRIVE AND MOTILITY (None □)						
80 Lack drive	□	□	□	□	□	□
81 Inhib. drive	□	□	□	□	□	□
82 Inc. drive	□	□	□	□	□	□
83 Motr. restless.	□	□	□	□	□	□
84 Parakinesia	□	□	□	□	□	□
85 Mannerisms	□	□	□	□	□	□
86 Histrionic	□	□	□	□	□	□
87 Mutism	□	□	□	□	□	□
88 Logorrhea	□	□	□	□	□	□
CIRCADIAN DISTURBANCES (None □)						
89 Worse AM	□	□	□	□	□	□
90 Worse PM	□	□	□	□	□	□
91 Better PM	□	□	□	□	□	□
OTHER DISTURBANCES (None □)						
92 Soc. withdrawal	□	□	□	□	□	□
93 Exc. soc. contact	□	□	□	□	□	□
94 Aggressive	□	□	□	□	□	□
95 Suicide	□	□	□	□	□	□
96 Self-mutilation	□	□	□	□	□	□
97 Lack. feel. ill	□	□	□	□	□	□
98 Lack insight	□	□	□	□	□	□
99 Uncooperative	□	□	□	□	□	□
100 Lack self care	□	□	□	□	□	□
OTHER SYMPTOMS (None □)						
P1 Loss desire live	□	□	□	□	□	□
P2 Asthenia	□	□	□	□	□	□
P3 Accel. thinking	□	□	□	□	□	□
P4 Tension	□	□	□	□	□	□
P5 Inc. libido	□	□	□	□	□	□
P6 Sex dysfunction	□	□	□	□	□	□
P7 Altered sexuality	□	□	□	□	□	□
P8 Thought echo	□	□	□	□	□	□
P9 Pseudohalluc.	□	□	□	□	□	□
P10 ________	□	□	□	□	□	□
P11 ________	□	□	□	□	□	□
P12 ________	□	□	□	□	□	□
P13 ________	□	□	□	□	□	□
P14 ________	□	□	□	□	□	□
P15 ________	□	□	□	□	□	□
Unreliability	□	□	□	□	□	
	AB 0	MI 1	MO 2	SV 3	EX 4	NA (9)

HOSPITAL/CLINIC:

RATER:

SOMATIC SIGNS
AMDP - 5

PATIENT INITIALS ___ ___ (1st Last) PT. NO.________

SEX: M____ F____

BIRTH DATE:________

RAGE: W__ B__ I__ O__ OTH________

DATE OF EXAMINATION: ___/___/___ (M D Y)

Patient Number
Study Number
Sex (M = 1; F = 2)
Age
Race (W=1, B=2, I=3, O=4, Oth =5)
Date of Examination (M D Y)
Period

Rating scale: 0 AB, 1 MI, 2 MO, 3 SV, 4 EX, (9) NA

SLEEP/VIGILANCE DISTURBANCES (None ☐)
101 Diff. fall. asleep
102 Interrupted sleep
103 Shortened sleep
104 Early wakening
105 Drowsiness

APPETITE DISTURBANCES (None ☐)
106 Decr. appetite
107 Inc. appetite
108 Exc. thirst
109 Decr. libido

G.I. DISTURBANCES (None ☐)
110 Hypersalivation
111 Dry mouth
112 Nausea
113 Vomiting
114 Gastric discomfort
115 Constipation
116 Diarrhea

CARDIO-RESPIRATORY DISTURBANCES (None ☐)
117 Breathing diff.
118 Dizziness
119 Palpitations
120 Cardiac pain

AUTONOMIC DISTURBANCES (None ☐)
121 Blurred vision
122 Inc. perspiration
123 Seborrhea
124 Micturition diff.
125 Menstrual diff.

OTHER SOMATIC DISTURBANCES (None ☐)
126 Headache
127 Backache
128 Heaviness in legs
129 Hot flashes
130 Chills
131 Conversion symptoms

NEUROLOGICAL DISTURBANCES (None ☐)
132 Hypertonia
133 Hypotonia
134 Tremor
135 Acute dyskinesia
136 Hypokinesia
137 Akathisia
138 Ataxia
139 Nystagmus
140 Paresthesia

OTHER SYMPTOMS (None ☐)
S1 Dreams/Nightmares
S2 Allergic reactions
S3 Tardive dyskinesia
S4 Dependent edema
S5 ______
S6 ______
S7 ______

Laterality N ☐ Y ☐
Convulsions N ☐ Y ☐

Weight (lbs)
Temperature (^{o}F)
Pulse (/mn)
BP, sitting, dia.
BP, sitting, sys.
BP, standing, dia.
BP, standing, sys.

STANDARD SOMATIC INQUIRY (from the French AMDP)

How have you been feeling physically in the last few days? Sleeping well? (101-104) Bothered by dreams/nightmares? (S1) Sleeping during the day? (105)
Appetite good? (106,107) Drinking more water than usual? (108,111)
Problems with digestion? Changes in defecation or urination from normal? (112-116, 124)
Difficulty breathing? (117) Dizziness? (118) Blurred vision? (121)
Heart pounding or beating faster? (119,120)
Legs feel heavy? (128) Ankles swelling? (87)
Feeling warm (hot flashes)? (129) Chills? (130) Perspiring (sweating more than usual? (122) Problems with skin (rash)? (23,S2)
Any aches or pains? (114,126,127) Any tingling? (140)
Periods regular? (135) Sexual difficulties (frigidity, ejaculation)? (109)
Any other physical symptoms or signs?

COMMENTS

病院（施設）名：
評価者氏名：
研究課題（番号）：

AMDP - 4

患 者 氏 名：
性 別：
生 年 月 日：
診 断 名：
評価実施年月日：
観察期間（日）：

患者記録番号
現試験期間中の患者番号
性 （男＝1；女＝2）
年令
ICD－9診断分類
評価実施年月日
評価日ナンバー

0	1	2	3	4	(5)
無	軽度	中等度	重度	極重度	

意識障害
1 意識減弱
2 意識混沌
3 意識狭縮
4 意識変移

見当識障害
5 時 間 的
6 場 所 的
7 状 況
8 自己に関する

注意力・記憶の障害
9 把握障害
10 集中障害
11 記銘障害
12 記憶障害
13 作 話
14 記憶錯誤

形式的思考障害
15 制 止
16 緩 徐
17 迂 遠
18 狭 小
19 保 続
20 詮索（思い悩む）
21 思考促迫
22 観念奔逸
23 的はずれ応答
24 途絶／思考断絶
25 散乱／支離滅裂
26 造 語 症

恐れ・強迫
27 不 信
28 心 気 症
29 恐 怖 症
30 強迫思考
31 強迫衝動
32 強迫行為

妄 想
33 妄想気分
34 妄想知覚
35 妄想着想
36 妄想思考
37 体系化された妄想
38 妄想力動
39 関係妄想
40 被害・迫害妄想
41 嫉妬妄想
42 罪責妄想
43 貧困妄想
44 心気妄想
45 誇大妄想
46 その他の妄想

感覚錯誤
47 錯 覚
48 幻声（音声幻覚）
49 その他の聴覚幻覚(要素幻聴)
50 視覚幻覚
51 体感幻覚
52 幻嗅幻味

自我障害
53 現実感喪失
54 離人症
55 考想伝播
56 思考奪取
57 思考吹入
58 他の外的被影響体験

情動性の障害
59 困 惑
60 無感情感
61 情動貧困
62 生気感情の障害
63 意気沮喪
64 絶 望
65 不 安
66 多 幸 感
67 不 快 感
68 いらだち
69 内的不穏
70 悲嘆／悲哀
71 不 全 感
72 自己価値感情高揚
73 罪 責 感
74 貧 困 感
75 両 価 性
76 気分倒錯
77 情動不安定
78 情動失禁
79 情動硬直

発動性，精神運動性障害
80 発動性貧困
81 発動性制止
82 発動性高揚
83 運動性不穏
84 運動錯誤
85 衒奇／奇異
86 芝居がかり（演技的）
87 緘黙（無言）
88 言葉洩れ

日内変動
89 午前悪化
90 午後悪化
91 午後軽快

その他の障害
92 社会的退却
93 社会的活動性
94 攻 撃 性
95 自 殺 性
96 自 傷
97 病感欠如
98 病識欠如
99 治療拒否
100 看護の必要度

P1
P2
P3
P4
P5
P6
P7
P8
P9
P10
P11
P12
P13
P14
P15

0	1	2	3	4	(5)

病院（施設）名：
評価者氏名：
研究課題（番号）：

AMDP - 5

患者氏名：...........................
....
性別：...........................
生年月日：...........................
診断名：...........................
....
評価実施年月日：...........................
観察期日（日）：...........................

└┴┴┴┴┴┴┴┘	患者の記録番号
└┴┴┴┴┘	現試験期間中の患者番号
└┘	性（男＝１；女＝２）
└┴┘	年令
└┴┴┴┴┘	ＩＣＤ－9診断分類
└┴┴┴┴┴┴┴┘	評価実施年月日
└┴┘	評価日ナンバー

□ 睡眠・覚醒障害

	0 無	1 軽度	2 中等度	3 重度	4 極重度	(5)
101 入眠障害	□	□	□	□	□	□
102 睡眠持続障害	□	□	□	□	□	□
103 睡眠時間短縮	□	□	□	□	□	□
104 早期覚醒	□	□	□	□	□	□
105 倦怠	□	□	□	□	□	□

□ 食欲障害

	0 無	1 軽度	2 中等度	3 重度	4 極重度	(5)
106 食欲減退	□	□	□	□	□	□
107 食欲亢進	□	□	□	□	□	□
108 渇感亢進	□	□	□	□	□	□
109 性欲減退	□	□	□	□	□	□

□ 胃腸障害

	0 無	1 軽度	2 中等度	3 重度	4 極重度	(5)
110 流涎過多	□	□	□	□	□	□
111 口渇	□	□	□	□	□	□
112 悪心	□	□	□	□	□	□
113 嘔吐	□	□	□	□	□	□
114 胃の愁訴	□	□	□	□	□	□
115 便秘	□	□	□	□	□	□
116 下痢	□	□	□	□	□	□

□ 心臓・呼吸器系障害

	0 無	1 軽度	2 中等度	3 重度	4 極重度	(5)
117 呼吸愁訴	□	□	□	□	□	□
118 めまい	□	□	□	□	□	□
119 動悸	□	□	□	□	□	□
120 心臓圧迫感	□	□	□	□	□	□

□ その他の自律神経障害

	0 無	1 軽度	2 中等度	3 重度	4 極重度	(5)
121 輻輳調節障害	□	□	□	□	□	□
122 発汗亢進	□	□	□	□	□	□
123 脂漏	□	□	□	□	□	□
124 排尿障害	□	□	□	□	□	□
125 月経障害	□	□	□	□	□	□

□ その他の障害

	0 無	1 軽度	2 中等度	3 重度	4 極重度	(5)
126 頭重	□	□	□	□	□	□
127 背部愁訴	□	□	□	□	□	□
128 脚部重感	□	□	□	□	□	□
129 熱感	□	□	□	□	□	□
130 悪寒	□	□	□	□	□	□
131 転換症状	□	□	□	□	□	□

□ 神経学的障害

	0 無	1 軽度	2 中等度	3 重度	4 極重度	(5)
132 硬直（強剛）	□	□	□	□	□	□
133 筋緊張低下	□	□	□	□	□	□
134 振せん	□	□	□	□	□	□
135 ジスキネジー	□	□	□	□	□	□
136 運動減少症	□	□	□	□	□	□
137 アカシジア	□	□	□	□	□	□
138 運動失調症	□	□	□	□	□	□
139 眼振	□	□	□	□	□	□
140 錯感覚	□	□	□	□	□	□

□

	0 無	1 軽度	2 中等度	3 重度	4 極重度	(5)
S1	□	□	□	□	□	□
S2	□	□	□	□	□	□
S3	□	□	□	□	□	□
S4	□	□	□	□	□	□
S5	□	□	□	□	□	□
S6	□	□	□	□	□	□
S7	□	□	□	□	□	□

体側による差 □ □
痙攣発作 □ □

└┴┴┘ (ex.: 036)
└┴┴┘ (ex.: 374)
└┴┴┘ (ex.: 072)
└┴┴┘ (ex.: 135)
└┴┴┘ (ex.: 080)
└┴┴┘
└┴┴┘

Hospital/klinik

Rater:

PSYKOPATOLOGISKE SYMPTOMER

AMDP - 4

Patientnummer

Undersøgelsesnummer

Køn (mand = 1, kvinde = 2)

Alder

Dato for undersøgelsen

Periode

Rating scale: 0 ikke til stede · 1 let · 2 middel · 3 svær · 4 extr. · (5) ej vb.

Bevidsthedsforstyrrelser

1 Bevidsthedssvækkelse
2 Bevidsthedsplumring
3 Bevidsthedsindsnævring
4 Bevidsthedsudvidelse'

Forstyrrelser i orienteringsevnen

5 Tid
6 Sted
7 Situation
8 Egne data

Opmærksomheds- og hukommelsesforstyrrelser

9 Apperceptionsforstyrrelser
10 Koncentrationsforstyrrelser'
11 Forstyr. af korttidshukom.
12 Retentionsforstyrrelser
13 Konfabulationer
14 Hukommelsesforskydning

Formelle tankeforstyrrelser

15 Tankehæmning (subj.)
16 Tankehæmning (obs.)
17 Omstænd. i tankegang
18 Persever. i tankegang
19 Verbal perseveration
20 Grublen
21 Komprimeret tankegang
22 Tankeflugt
23 Tangentiel tankegang
24 Tankespærring
25 Inkoherænt tankegang
26 Neologismer

Tvangstanker/handlinger

27 Mistænksomhed
28 Non-paranoid hypokondri
29 Fobier
30 Tvangstanker
31 Tvangsimpulser
32 Tvangshandlinger

Vrangforestillinger

33 Primær paranoid affekt
34 Paranoide percept.fortolkn.
35 Paranoide indfald
36 Usystem. vrangforestil.
37 System. vrangforestil.
38 Sekundær paranoid affekt
39 Selvhenførende forestil.
40 Forfølgelses forestil.
41 Jalousiforestillinger
42 Skyldforestillinger
43 Forarmelsesforestillinger
44 Hypokondre forestillinger
45 Storhedsforestillinger
46 Andre vrangforestillinger

Perceptionsforstyrrelser

47 Illusioner
48 Verbale hallucinationer
49 Andre hørehallucinationer
50 Synshallucinationer
51 Følehallucinationer
52 Lugt- og smagshallucinat.

Jeg-forstyrrelser

53 Derealisation
54 Depersonalisation
55 Tankehørlighed
56 Tanketyveri
57 Tankepåvirkning
58 Andre påvirkn.fænomener

Affektive forstyrrelser

59 Rådvildhed
60 Mgl.reaktivitet (rapp.)
61 Mgl.reaktivitet (obs.)
62 Mgl. vitalitet
63 Forsænket stemningsleje
64 Håbløshed
65 Angst, psykisk
66 Løftet stemningsleje
67 Dysfori
68 Irritabilitet
69 Indre uro
70 Klagende adfærd
71 Selvundervurdering
72 Selvovervurdering
73 Skyldfølelse
74 Oplevelse af forarmelse
75 Ambivalens
76 Paratymi
77 Affektlabilitet
78 Affektinkontinens
79 Affektrigiditet

Forstyrrelser i initiativ og psykomotorik

80 Psykomotorik, nedsat
81 Initiativ, nedsat
82 Initiativ, øget
83 Psykomotorik, øget

84 Parakinesi
85 Bizar adfærd
86 Teatralsk adfærd
87 Mutisme
88 Logorré

Circadiane svingninger

89 Morgen værst
90 Aften værst
91 Aftenbedring

Andre forstyrrelser

92 Nedsat social kontakt
93 Overdreven social kontakt
94 Aggressivitet
95 Suicidale impulser
96 Selvmutilation
97 Mgl. sygdomsfornemmelse
98 Mgl. sygdomsindsigt
99 Behandlingsvægring
100 Mgl. selvhjulpethed

P1 Depressionens kvalitet
P2 Persistens
P3 Motorisk tension
P4 Anklager andre
P5 Arbejdsevne, nedsat
P6 Arbejdsevne, øget
P7 Verbal aktivitet nedsat
P8 Verbal aktivitet øget
P9 Asteni
P10 Højrøstethed
P11
P12
P13
P14
P15

Hospital/klinik

Rater:

SOMATISKE SYMPTOMER

AMDP - 5

Patient nummer

Undersøgelsesnummer

Køn (mand = 1, kvinde = 2)

Alder

Dato for undersøgelsen

Periode

Scale (each column): 0 ikke til stede, 1 let, 2 middel, 3 svær, 4 extr., (5) ej vb.

Søvnforstyrrelser

101 Indsovningsbesvær
102 Afbrudt søvn
103 Nedsat søvnlængde
104 Tidlig morgenvågning
105 Søvnighed

Forstyrrelse af appetit og sexuel interesse

106 Nedsat appetit
107 Øget appetit
108 Øget tørst
109 Nedsat sexuel interesse

Gastro-intestinale forstyrrelser

110 Øget spytsekretion
111 Mundtørhed
112 Kvalme
113 Opkastninger
114 Dyspepsi
115 Obstipation
116 Diaré

Kardio-respiratoriske forstyrrelser

117 Åndedrætsbesvær
118 Svimmelhed
119 Hjertebanken
120 Hjertesmerter

Andre vegetative forstyrrelser

121 Akkomodationsforstyr.
122 Øget perspiration
123 Seboré
124 Miktionsforstyrrelser
125 Menstruationsforstyr.

Andre forstyrrelser

126 Hovedpine
127 Rygsmerter
128 Tyngdefølelse i benene
129 Varmefornemmelser
130 Kuldegysninger
131 Konversionssymptomer

Neurologiske forstyrrelser

132 Rigiditet
133 Nedsat muskeltonus
134 Tremor
135 Dyskinesi, akut
136 Hypokinesi
137 Akatisi
138 Ataksi
139 Nystagmus
140 Paræstesi

S1 Vægttab
S2 Vægtøgning
S3 Øget sexuel interesse
S4 Dyskinesi, tardiv
S5 Epileptisk anfald
S6 Øget drømmeaktivitet
S7 Allergisk reaktion

(ex.: 036)
(ex.: 374)
(ex.: 072)
(ex.: 135)
(ex.: 080)

ΙΔΡΥΜΑ:

ΕΞΕΤΑΣΤΗΣ:

ΚΛΙΜΑΚΑ ΨΥΧΟΠΑΘΟΛΟΓΙΑΣ
AMDP - 4

Ονοματεπώνυμο ασθενούς ....

Φύλο ....

Ημερομηνία γέννησης ....

Διάγνωση ....

Ημερομηνία εξέτασης ....

Περίοδος εκτίμησης (σε μέρες) ....

Αρ. φακέλλου τού ασθενούς

Αρ. τού ασθενούς στη μελέτη

Φύλο (Άνδρας=1, Γυναίκα=2)

Ηλικία

Διάγνωση ICD 9

Ημερομηνία εξέτασης

Αριθμός ημερών που εκτιμήθηκαν

Ημερομηνία εγγραφής σε video:

Ρυθμιστής:

0	1	2	3	4	(5)
απουσιάζει	ελαφρύ	μέτριο	ισχυρό	πολύ ισχυρό	χωρίς γνώμη

Διαταραχές της συνείδησης (καμιά)

1 Μείωση εγρήγορσης
2 Θόλωση συνείδησης
3 Στένωση πεδίου συνείδησης
4 Διεύρυνση συνείδησης

Διαταραχές του προσανατολισμού (καμιά)

5 Δ.Π. ως προς το χρόνο
6 Δ.Π. ως προς τον τόπο
7 Δ.Π. ως προς την παρούσα συνθήκη
8 Δ.Π. ως προς τον εαυτό

Διαταραχές προσοχής και μνήμης (καμιά)

9 Δ. σημασιολόγησης της αντίληψης
10 Δ. συγκέντρωσης
11 Δ. απομνημόνευσης
12 Δ. ανάκλησης
13 Μυθοπλασία
14 Παραμνησίες/υπερμνησίες

Διαταραχές της σκέψης (καμιά)

15 Ανεσταλμένη σκέψη
16 Επιβράδυνση σκέψης
17 Παρεκλίνουσα σκέψη
18 Φτωχή σκέψη
19 Λεκτική εμμονή
20 Μυρικασμός
21 Αυτοματική σκέψη
22 Ιδεοφυγή
23 Παράπλευρες απαντήσεις
24 Ανακοπή σκέψης
25 Ασυνάρτητη σκέψη
26 Νεολογισμοί

απουσιάζει	ελαφρύ	μέτριο	ισχυρό	πολύ ισχυρό	χωρίς γνώμη
0	1	2	3	4	(5)

0	1	2	3	4	(5)
απουσιάζει	ελαφρύ	μέτριο	ισχυρό	πολύ ισχυρό	χωρίς γνώμη

Φοβίες και ιδεοληψίες (καμιά)

27 Δυσπιστία
28 Μη παραληρητική υποχονδρία
29 Φοβίες
30 Ιδεοληψίες
31 Ιδεοληψίες-Παρορμήσεις
32 Ψυχαναγκασμοί

Παραλήρημα (κανένα)

33 Παραληρητικό προαίσθημα
34 Παραληρητική αντίληψη
35 Παραληρητική διαίσθηση
36 Μη συστ/μένες παραληρητικές ιδέες
37 Συστηματοποιημένο παραλήρημα
38 Δυναμισμός παραληρήματος
39 Παραληρητικές ιδέες αυτοαναφοράς
40 Παραληρητικές ιδέες καταδίωξης
41 Παραληρητικές ιδέες ζηλοτυπίας
42 Παραληρητικές ιδέες ενοχής
43 Παραληρητικές ιδέες καταστροφής
44 Υποχονδριακές παραληρητικές ιδέες
45 Παραληρητικές ιδέες μεγαλείου
46 Φανταστικές παραληρητικές ιδέες

Διαταραχές της αντίληψης (καμιά)

47 Παραισθήσεις
48 Ακουστικολεκτικές ψευδαισθήσεις
49 Άλλες ακουστικές ψευδαισθήσεις
50 Οπτικές ψευδαισθήσεις
51 Κοιναισθητικές ψευδαισθησεις
52 Οσφρητικές & γευστ. ψευδαισθήσεις

απουσιάζει	ελαφρύ	μέτριο	ισχυρό	πολύ ισχυρό	χωρίς γνώμη
0	1	2	3	4	(5)

0	1	2	3	4	(5)
απουσιάζει	ελαφρύ	μέτριο	ισχυρό	πολύ ισχυρό	χωρίς γνώμη

Διαταραχές του εγώ (καμιά)

53 Αποπραγματοποίηση
54 Αποπροσωποποίηση
55 Ανάγνωση σκέψης
56 Υφαρπαγή σκέψης
57 Επιβεβλημένες σκέψεις
58 Άλλες ιδέες επίδρασης

Διαταραχές του συναισθήματος (καμιά)

59 Αμηχανία
60 Συναισθ. απώλειας συναισθήματος
61 Συναισθηματική μείωση
62 Δ. συναισθήματος ζωτικότητας
63 Καταθλιπτικό συναίσθημα
64 Απελπισία
65 Άγχος
66 Ευφορία
67 Δυσφορία
68 Ευερεθιστότητα
69 Εσωτερική ανησυχία
70 Τάση για μεμψιμοιρία
71 Συναίσθημα ανεπάρκειας
72 Υπερτίμηση εαυτού
73 Συναίσθημα ενοχής
74 Συναίσθημα καταστροφής
75 Συναισθηματική αμφιθυμία
76 Συναισθηματική δυσαρμονία
77 Συναισθηματική ευμεταβλητότητα
78 Υπερευσυγκινησία
79 Συναισθηματική μονοτονία

Διαταραχές της ζωικής ορμής και ψυχοκινητικότητας (καμιά)

80 Μείωση ενεργητικότητας
81 Αναστολή ενεργητικότητας
82 Αύξηση ενεργητικότητας
83 Κινητική ανησυχία

Δυσκολία εκτίμησης

απουσιάζει	ελαφρύ	μέτριο	ισχυρό	πολύ ισχυρό	χωρίς γνώμη
0	1	2	3	4	(5)

0	1	2	3	4	(5)
απουσιάζει	ελαφρύ	μέτριο	ισχυρό	πολύ ισχυρό	χωρίς γνώμη

84 Παρακινησίες
85 Μανιερισμοί/ιδιοτροπισμοί
86 Οιστριονισμός
87 Λακωνισμός
88 Λογόρροια

Δ/χές νυχθημερήσιου κύκλου (καμιά)

89 Πρωινή επιδείνωση
90 Εσπερινή επιδείνωση
91 Εσπερινή βελτίωση

Άλλες ψυχοπαθολογικές Δ/χές (καμιά)

92 Μειωμένη κοινωνικότητα
93 Υπερβολική κοινωνικότητα
94 Επιθετικότητα
95 Αυτοκτονικές τάσεις
96 Αυτοτραυματισμοί
97 Άρνηση νοσηρού
98 Απουσία εναισθησίας
99 Άρνηση θεραπείας
100 Ανάγκη φροντίδας

Εφεδρικά ψυχοπαθ/κά συμπτώματα (κανένα)

P1 Μη παραληρητική μυθοπλασία
P2 Απώλεια επιθυμίας ζωής
P3 Ασθενική κατάσταση
P4 Επιτάχυνση σκέψης
P5 Υπερένταση
P6 Τάση δραματοποίησης
P7 Αγχώδης προσμονή
P8 Άγχος κοινωνικών περιστάσεων
P9 Έκδηλο άγχος
P10 Μειωμένη σεξουαλική επιθυμία
P11 Οξυμένη σεξουαλική επιθυμία
P12 Σεξουαλική ανηδονία
P13 Σεξουαλικές αποκλίσεις
P14 Ψευδοψευδαισθήσεις
P15 Κοινωνική αναπηρία

απουσιάζει	ελαφρύ	μέτριο	ισχυρό	πολύ ισχυρό	χωρίς γνώμη
0	1	2	3	4	(5)

ΙΔΡΥΜΑ:

ΕΞΕΤΑΣΤΗΣ:

ΣΩΜΑΤΙΚΗ ΚΛΙΜΑΚΑ
AMDP - 5

Ονοματεπώνυμο ασθενούς	Αρ. φακέλλου τού ασθενούς
....	Αρ. τού ασθενούς στη μελέτη
Φύλο :	Φύλο (Άνδρας=1, Γυναίκα=2)
Ημερομηνία γέννησης	Ηλικία
Διάγνωση	Διάγνωση ICD 9
....	
Ημερομηνία εξέτασης	Ημερομηνία εξέτασης
Περίοδος εκτίμησης (σε μέρες)	Αριθμός ημερών που εκτιμήθηκαν

Διαταραχές ύπνου και επιπέδου εγρήγορσης (καμιά □)

	0 απουσιάζει	1 ελαφρύ	2 μέτριο	3 ισχυρό	4 πολύ ισχυρό	(5) χωρίς γνώμη
101 Δυσκολίες επέλευσης ύπνου	□	□	□	□	□	□
102 Νυχτ. αφύπνιση ή διακ/μενος ύπνος	□	□	□	□	□	□
103 Μειωμένη διάρκεια ύπνου	□	□	□	□	□	□
104 Πρώιμη αφύπνιση	□	□	□	□	□	□
105 Υπνηλία	□	□	□	□	□	□

Διαταραχές επιθυμιών (καμιά □)

	0	1	2	3	4	(5)
106 Μειωμένη όρεξη	□	□	□	□	□	□
107 Αυξημένη όρεξη	□	□	□	□	□	□
108 Αυξημένη δίψα	□	□	□	□	□	□
109 Ανικανότητα/ψυχρότητα	□	□	□	□	□	□

Γαστροεντερικές διαταραχές (καμιά □)

	0	1	2	3	4	(5)
110 Υπερέκκριση σάλιου	□	□	□	□	□	□
111 Στοματική ξηρότητα	□	□	□	□	□	□
112 Ναυτίες	□	□	□	□	□	□
113 Εμμετοί	□	□	□	□	□	□
114 Γαστρικά ενοχλήματα	□	□	□	□	□	□
115 Δυσκοιλιότητα	□	□	□	□	□	□
116 Διάρροια	□	□	□	□	□	□

Καρδιοαναπνευστικές διαταραχές (καμιά □)

	0 απουσιάζει	1 ελαφρύ	2 μέτριο	3 ισχυρό	4 πολύ ισχυρό	(5) χωρίς γνώμη
117 Δυσκολία αναπνοής	□	□	□	□	□	□
118 Ίλιγγοι	□	□	□	□	□	□
119 Ταχυπαλμίες	□	□	□	□	□	□
120 Προκάρδια άλγη	□	□	□	□	□	□

Άλλες νευροφυτικές διαταραχές (καμιά □)

	0	1	2	3	4	(5)
121 Διαταραχές προσαρμοστότητας	□	□	□	□	□	□
122 Αυξημένη εφίδρωση	□	□	□	□	□	□
123 Σμηγματόρροια	□	□	□	□	□	□
124 Δυσκολία ούρησης	□	□	□	□	□	□
125 Διαταραχές εμμήνων	□	□	□	□	□	□

Άλλες σωματικές διαταραχές (καμιά □)

	0	1	2	3	4	(5)
126 Ενοχλήματα στο κεφάλι	□	□	□	□	□	□
127 Οσφυαλγίες/ραχιαλγίες	□	□	□	□	□	□
128 Βάρος μηρών	□	□	□	□	□	□
129 Αίσθημα ζέστης	□	□	□	□	□	□
130 Κρυάδες	□	□	□	□	□	□
131 Συμπτώματα μετατροπής	□	□	□	□	□	□

Νευρολογικές διαταραχές (καμιά □)

	0 απουσιάζει	1 ελαφρύ	2 μέτριο	3 ισχυρό	4 πολύ ισχυρό	(5) χωρίς γνώμη
132 Υπερτονία	□	□	□	□	□	□
133 Υποτονία	□	□	□	□	□	□
134 Τρόμος	□	□	□	□	□	□
135 Δυσκινησία	□	□	□	□	□	□
136 Υποκινησία/υπομιμία	□	□	□	□	□	□
137 Ακαθησία	□	□	□	□	□	□
138 Αταξία	□	□	□	□	□	□
139 Νυσταγμός	□	□	□	□	□	□
140 Παραισθησίες	□	□	□	□	□	□

Εφεδρικά σωματικά συμπτώματα (κανένα □)

	0 απουσιάζει	1 ελαφρύ	2 μέτριο	3 ισχυρό	4 πολύ ισχυρό	(5) χωρίς γνώμη
S1 Σωματικό άγχος	□	□	□	□	□	□
S2 Όνειρα/εφιάλτες	□	□	□	□	□	□
S3 Καθυστερημένη εκσπερμάτωση	□	□	□	□	□	□
S4 Αλλεργικές αντιδράσεις	□	□	□	□	□	□
S5 Τικς/βαταρισμός	□	□	□	□	□	□
S6 Όψιμη δυσκινησία	□	□	□	□	□	□
S7 Σφυραία οιδήματα	□	□	□	□	□	□

Νευρ/κή ασυμ.	Όχι □	Ναί □
Επιληπτ. κρίση	Όχι □	Ναί □

ΜΕΤΡΗΣΕΙΣ

βάρος (χλγ)		(π.χ.: 036)
θερμοκρασία (°C)		(π.χ.: 374)
σφυγμός (/λεπτ.)		(π.χ.: 072)
ΑΠ ξαπλωμένος, μέγ. (mm Hg)		(π.χ.: 135)
ΑΠ ξαπλωμένος, ελάχ. (mm Hg)		(π.χ.: 080)
ΑΠ όρθιος, μέγ. (mm Hg)		
ΑΠ όρθιος, ελάχ. (mm Hg)		

ΠΑΡΑΤΗΡΗΣΕΙΣ

INSTITUIÇÃO:
OBSERVADOR:

ESCALA PSICOPATOLÓGICA AMDP - 4

Nome do DOENTE	└┴┴┴┴┴┘	N.° do processo do doente
....	└┴┴┴┘	N.° do doente no estudo
SEXO:	└┘	Sexo (M=1; F=2)
DATA DE NASCIMENTO	└┴┘	Idade
DIAGNÓSTICO	└┴┴┴┘	Diagnóstico CID-9
....		
DATA DA OBSERVAÇÃO	└┴┴┴┴┴┘	Data da observação
PERÍODO AVALIADO (dias)	└┴┘	Número de dias avaliados

DATA DA COTAÇÃO VIDEO eventual:
MODERADOR:

Escala: 0 ausente — 1 ligeiro — 2 moderado — 3 intenso — 4 muito intenso — (5) sem opinião

Perturbações da consciência (nada □)
1 Diminuição da vigilidade
2 Turvação da consciência
3 Estreitamento da consciência
4 Expansão da consciência

Perturbações da orientação (nada □)
5 No tempo
6 No espaço
7 Relativas à situação
8 Relativas à própria pessoa

Perturbações da atenção e da memória (nada □)
9 Perturbações da apreensão
10 Perturbações da concentração
11 Perturbações da memorização
12 Perturbações da evocação
13 Confabulação
14 Paramenésias/Hipermnésias

Perturbações formais do pensamento (nada □)
15 Pensamento inibido
16 Pensamento lentificado
17 Pensamento circunstanciado
18 Pobreza do pensamento
19 Perseveração verbal
20 Ruminação (não obsessiva)
21 Pensamento automático
22 Fuga de ideias
23 Respostas ao lado
24 Pensamento bloqueado
25 Pensamento desagregado/incoerente
26 Neologismos

Temores e obsessões (nada □)
27 Desconfiança
28 Hipocondria (não delirante)
29 Fobias
30 Pensamentos obsessivos
31 Impulsos obsessivos
32 Compulsões

Delírio (nada □)
33 Humor delirante
34 Percepção delirante
35 Intuição delirante
36 Ideias delirantes não sistematizadas
37 Delírio sistematizado
38 Dinamismo do delírio
39 Auto-relacionação delirante
40 I. D. de prejuízo/perseguição
41 I.D. de ciúme
42 I.D. de culpabilidade
43 I.D. de ruina
44 I.D. de hipocondríacas
45 I.D. de grandeza
46 Outros temas delirantes

Perturbações psico-sensoriais (nada □)
47 Ilusões
48 Alucinações acustico-verbais
49 Outras alucinações auditivas
50 Alucinações visuais
51 Alucinações cenestésicas
52 Alucinações olfact. e gustativas

Perturbações da vivência do eu (nada □)
53 Desrealização
54 Despersonalização
55 Difusão do pensamento
56 Roubo do pensamento
57 Influenciamento do pensamento
58 Outras vivências de influenciamento

Perturbações da afectividade (nada □)
59 Perplexidade
60 Anestesia afectiva
61 Indiferença afectiva
62 Perturbações dos afectos vitais
63 Tristeza (humor depressivo)
64 Pessimismo
65 Ansiedade (psíquica)
66 Euforia
67 Disforia
68 Irritabilidade
69 Agitação interior
70 Propensão a queixar-se
71 Sentimentos de auto-desvalorização
72 Sentimentos de sobrevalorização
73 Sentimentos de culpa
74 Sentimentos de ruina
75 Ambivalência afectiva
76 Discordância afectiva
77 Labilidade afectiva
78 Incontinência afectiva
79 Rigidez afectiva

Perturbações de energia vital e da psicomotrocidade (nada □)
80 Diminuição da energia
81 Inibição da energia
82 Aumento da energia
83 Agitação psicomotora
84 Paracinésias
85 Maneirismos/bizarrias
86 Teatralidade
87 Laconismo
88 Logorreia

Variações circadianas (nada □)
89 Agravamento matinal
90 Agravamento vesperal
91 Melhoria vesperal

Outras perturbações psicopatológicas (nada □)
92 Diminuição da sociabilidade
93 Sociabilidade exagerada
94 Agressividade
95 Tendências suicidas
96 Auto-agressões
97 Ausência de sent. de estar doente
98 Ausência de crítica da doença
99 Recusa de tratamento
100 Necessidade de cuidados

Items psicopat. de reserva (nada □)
P1 Fabulação (não delirante)
P2 Perda do gosto de viver
P3 Astenia
P4 Pensamento acelerado
P5 Tensão
P6 Tendência a dramatizar
P7 Antecipação ansiosa
P8 Ansiedade social
P9 Comportamento ansioso
P10 Diminuição da libido
P11 Aumento da libido
P12 Insatisfação sexual
P13 Desvio sexual
P14 Alucinose
P15 Invalidação social

Dificuldade de avaliação

ausente 0 — ligeiro 1 — moderado 2 — intenso 3 — muito intenso 4 — sem opinião (5)

INSTITUIÇÃO:
OBSERVADOR:

ESCALA SOMÁTICA
AMDP - 5

Nome do DOENTE	└┴┴┴┴┴┘	N.° de processo do doente
....	└┴┴┴┘	N.° do doente no estudo
SEXO	└┘	Sexo (M=1; F=2)
DATA DE NASCIMENTO	└┴┘	Idade
DIAGNÓSTICO	└┴┴┴┘	Diagnóstico CID-9
....		
DATA DA OBSERVAÇÃO	└┴┴┴┴┴┘	Data da observação
PERÍODO AVALIADO (dias)	└┴┘	Número de dias avaliados

0	1	2	3	4	(5)
ausente	ligeiro	moderado	intenso	muito intenso	sem opinião

Perturbações do sono e da vigilidade
nada □

	0	1	2	3	4	(5)
101 Insónia inicial	□	□	□	□	□	□
102 Insónia intermediária	□	□	□	□	□	□
103 Dimininuição da duração do sono	□	□	□	□	□	□
104 Insónia matinal	□	□	□	□	□	□
105 Sonolência diurna	□	□	□	□	□	□

Perturbações do apetite
nada □

	0	1	2	3	4	(5)
106 Anorexia	□	□	□	□	□	□
107 Bulimia	□	□	□	□	□	□
108 Polidipsia	□	□	□	□	□	□
109 Impotência/frigidez	□	□	□	□	□	□

Perturbações gastro-intestinais
nada □

	0	1	2	3	4	(5)
110 Sialorreia	□	□	□	□	□	□
111 Secura da boca	□	□	□	□	□	□
112 Náuseas	□	□	□	□	□	□
113 Vómitos	□	□	□	□	□	□
114 Queixas gástricas	□	□	□	□	□	□
115 Obstipação	□	□	□	□	□	□
116 Diarreia	□	□	□	□	□	□

Perturbações cardio-respiratórias
nada □

	0	1	2	3	4	(5)
117 Dispneia	□	□	□	□	□	□
118 Vertigens	□	□	□	□	□	□
119 Palpitações	□	□	□	□	□	□
120 Precordialgias	□	□	□	□	□	□

Outras perturbações vegetativas
nada □

	0	1	2	3	4	(5)
121 Perturbações da acomodação	□	□	□	□	□	□
122 Diaforese	□	□	□	□	□	□
123 Seborreia	□	□	□	□	□	□
124 Disúria	□	□	□	□	□	□
125 Perturbações menstruais	□	□	□	□	□	□

Outras perturbações somáticas
nada □

	0	1	2	3	4	(5)
126 Queixas cefálicas	□	□	□	□	□	□
127 Lombalgias/dorsalgias	□	□	□	□	□	□
128 Sensação de pernas pesadas	□	□	□	□	□	□
129 Sensação de calor	□	□	□	□	□	□
130 Sensação de frio	□	□	□	□	□	□
131 Sintomas de conversão	□	□	□	□	□	□

Perturbações neurológicas
nada □

	0	1	2	3	4	(5)
132 Hipertonia	□	□	□	□	□	□
133 Hipotonia	□	□	□	□	□	□
134 Tremores	□	□	□	□	□	□
135 Crises discinéticas agudas	□	□	□	□	□	□
136 Hipocinésia/hipomimia	□	□	□	□	□	□
137 Acatisia/taquicinésia	□	□	□	□	□	□
138 Ataxia	□	□	□	□	□	□
139 Nistagmo	□	□	□	□	□	□
140 Parestesias	□	□	□	□	□	□

Items somáticos de reserva
nada □

	0	1	2	3	4	(5)
S1 Ansiedade somática	□	□	□	□	□	□
S2 Sonhos/pesadelos	□	□	□	□	□	□
S3 Ejaculação retardada	□	□	□	□	□	□
S4 Reacções alérgicas	□	□	□	□	□	□
S5 Tiques/gaguejar	□	□	□	□	□	□
S6 Discinésias tardias	□	□	□	□	□	□
S7 Edemas maleolares	□	□	□	□	□	□

Assim. neurol.	Não □	Sim □
Crises Epilépticas	Não □	Sim □

MEDIDAS:

Peso (Kg)	└─┴─┴─┘	(ex.: 036)
Temperatura (°C)	└─┴─┴─┘	(ex.: 374)
Pulso (/mn)	└─┴─┴─┘	(ex.: 072)
TA deitado, máx. (mmHg)	└─┴─┴─┘	(ex.: 135)
TA deitado, mín. (m/mHg)	└─┴─┴─┘	(ex.: 080)
TA em pé, máx. (m/mHg)	└─┴─┴─┘	
TA em pé, mín. (m/mHg)	└─┴─┴─┘	

ENTREVISTA SOMÁTICA ESTANDARDIZADA (F)

Como é que se sente fisicamente (nos últimos dias)?

Tem dormido bem? (101-104) Não tem sonhado? (S2) Não tem tido sono durante o dia? (105).

Tem tido bom apetite? (106-107) Tem bebido mais que habitualmente? (108-111).

Tem tido perturbações digestivas? Tem evacuado e urinado normalmente? (112-116, 124).

Tem tido dificuldade em em respirar? (117) Tem tido vertigens? (118) Tem tido a vista turva? (121).

O coração bate com muita força ou muito depressa? (119-120).

Tem sentido as pernas pesadas? Tem os tornozelos inchados? (128,S7).

Tem-se sentido anormalmente friorento ou encalorado? (129-130) Transpira mais do que de costume? (122) Tem tido borbulhas ou outras doenças da pele? (123,S4).

Não se sente bem em parte nenhuma? (114, 126, 127, S1) Tem sentido picadas? (140).

Segundo os casos: O período tem sido normal? (125) Notou a aparição duma frigidez/dificuldade de ejaculação? (109).

Tem mais algum sintoma físico a assinalar?

OBSERVAÇÕES INDIVIDUAIS

CENTRO:
EXAMINADOR:

ESCALA PSICOPATOLOGICA
AMDP - 4

APELLIDOS Y NOMBRE DEL ENFERMO: ....

SEXO: ....

FECHA DE NACIMIENTO: ....

DIAGNOSTICO: ....

FECHA DE LA EXPLORACION: ....

PERIODO CONSIDERADO (DIAS): ....

N.º DE HISTORIA DEL ENFERMO

N.º DEL ENFERMO EN ESTUDIO

SEXO (V = 1; H = 2)

EDAD

DIAGNOSTICO CIE-9

FECHA DE LA EXPLORACION

NUMERO DE DIAS EVALUADOS

FECHA DEL REGISTRO EN VIDEO EVENTUAL:

MODERADOR:

0	1	2	3	4	(5)
no tiene	li- gero	me- diano	in- tenso	muy intenso	Du- doso

ninguno ☐ TRASTORNOS DE CONCIENCIA
1 DISMINUCION CONCIENCIA
2 ENTURBAMIENTO DE LA C.
3 ESTRECHAMIENTO DE LA C.
4 EXPANSION/EXALTACION

ninguno ☐ TRASTORNOS DE LA ORIENTACION
5 DESOR. EN EL TIEMPO
6 D. EN EL ESPACIO
7 D. RESP. A LA SITUACION
8 D. RESP. PROPIA PERSONA

ninguno ☐ TRASTORNOS DE LA ATENCION Y DE LA MEMORIA
9 TR. DE LA APREHENSION
10 TR. DE LA CONCENTRACION
11 TR. DE LA FIJACION
12 HIPOAMNESIA
13 CONFABULACIONES
14 PARAMNESIAS/HIPERMNESIAS

ninguno ☐ TRASTORNOS FORMALES DE DEL PENSAMIENTO
15 INHIBICION DEL PENSAMIENTO
16 ENLENTECIMIENTO DEL PENS.
17 PENSAM. DIVAGATORIO
18 POBREZA DEL PENSAM.
19 PERSEVERACION DEL PENSAM.
20 RUMIACION
21 ACELERACION DEL PENSAM.
22 FUGA DE IDEAS
23 PARARRESPUESTAS
24 BLOQUEO INTERCEPT. DEL P.
25 P. DISGREGADO/INCOHERENTE
26 NEOLOGISMOS

ninguno ☐ TEMORES, ANANCASMOS
27 DESCONFIANZA (NO DELIR.)
28 HIPOCONDRIA (NO DELIR.)
29 FOBIAS
30 IDEAS OBSESIVAS
31 IMPULSOS OBSESIVOS
32 COMPULSIONES

ninguno ☐ DELIRIO (DELUSION)
33 HUMOR DELIRANTE
34 PERCEPCION DELIRANTE
35 INTUICION OCURRENCIA D.
36 IDEAS DELIRANTES
37 DELIRIO SISTEMATIZADO
38 DINAMICA (C. AFECT. DEL D.)
39 DELIRIO DE REFERENCIA
40 D. INFLUENCIA PERSECUCION
41 DELIRIO DE CELOS
42 DELIRIO DE CULPA
43 DELIRIO DE RUINA
44 DELIRIO HIPOCONDRIACO
45 DELIRIO DE GRANDEZA
46 OTROS CONT. DELIRANTES

ninguno ☐ TRASTORNOS DE LA SENSOPERCEPCION
47 ILUSIONES
48 OIR VOCES (FONEMAS)
49 OTRAS ALUC. ACUSTICAS
50 ALUCINACIONES OPTICAS
51 A. CENESTESICA CORPORALES
52 A. OLFATIVAS Y GUSTATIVAS

ninguno ☐ TRASTORNOS DE LA VIVENCIA DEL "YO"
53 DESREALIZACION
54 DESPERSONALIZACION
55 DIFUSION DEL PENSAMIENTO
56 ROBO, EXPROP. DEL PENSAM.
57 INFLUENCIA DEL PENSAM.
58 OTRAS VIVEN. DE INFLUENCIA

ninguno ☐ TRASTORNOS DE LA EFECTIVIDAD
59 PERPLEJIDAD
60 VIVENCIA DE VACIO AFECT.
61 EMPOBRECIMIENTO AFECTIVO
62 TRAST. SENTIM. VITALES
63 TRISTEZA, DEPRESION
64 DESESPERANZA
65 ANGUSTIA, ANSIEDAD
66 EUFORIA
67 DISFORIA
68 IRRITABILIDAD
69 INQUIETUD INTERNA
70 ACTITUD QUEJUMBROSA
71 SENTIM. DE INSUFICIENCIA
72 S. SOBREESTIMA DE SI MISMO
73 SENTIMIENTOS DE CULPA
74 SENTIMIENTOS DE RUINA
75 AMBIVALENCIA AFECTIVA
76 PARATIMIA (DISCOR. AFECT.)
77 LABILIDAD AFECTIVA
78 INCONTINENCIA AFECTIVA
79 RIGIDEZ AFECTIVA

ninguno ☐ TRASTORNOS DE LOS IMPULSOS Y DE LA PSICOMOTRICIDAD
80 POBREZA DE IMPULSOS
81 INHIBICION DE IMPULSOS
82 AUMENTO DE IMPULSIVIDAD
83 INQUIETUD PSICOMOTRIZ
84 PARAQUINESIAS
85 MANIERISMOS, AMANERAM.
86 TEATRALIDAD
87 MUTISMO
88 LOGORREA

ninguno ☐ VARIACIONES CIRCADIANAS
89 PEOR LAS PRIM. HORAS DIA
90 PEOR LAS ULT. HORAS DIA
91 MEJOR AL CAER LA TARDE

ninguno ☐ OTROS TRASTORNOS
92 DISMINU. DE LA SOCIABILIDAD
93 AUMENTO DE SOCIABILIDAD
94 AUMENTO DE AGRESIVIDAD
95 SUICIDALIDAD
96 AUTOAGRESIONES
97 FALTA DE SENS. DE ENFERM.
98 FALTA DE CONC. DE ENFERM.
99 RECHAZO DEL TRATAMIENTO
100 NECESIDAD DE CUIDADOS

☐ ITEM DE RESERVA
P1
P2
P3
P4
P5
P6
P7
P8
P9
P10
P11
P12
P13
P14
P15

INSEGURIDAD EN LOS HALLAZGOS DE LA EXPLORACION

no tiene	li- gero	me- diano	in- tenso	muy intenso	Du- doso
0	1	2	3	4	(5)

EXP. PSICOPATOLOGICA

TRASTORNOS DE LA CONCIENCIA

1. DISMINUCION DE LA CONCIENCIA
DUDOSO( ),NO( ),LIG.( ),MED.( ),INT.( )

2. ENTURBIAMIENTO DE LA CONCIENCIA
DUDOSO( ),NO( ),LIG.( ),MED.( ),INT.( )

3. ESTRECHAMIENTO DE LA CONCIENCIA
DUDOSO( ),NO( ),LIG.( ),MED.( ),INT.( )

4. EXALTACION DE LA CONCIENCIA
DUDOSO( ),NO( ),LIG.( ),MED.( ),INT.( )

TRASTORNOS DE LA ORIENTACION

5. DESORIENTACION TEMPORAL
DUDOSO( ),NO( ),LIG.( ),MED.( ),INT.( )

6. DESORIENTACION ESPACIAL
DUDOSO( ),NO( ),LIG.( ),MED.( ),INT.( )

7. DESORIENTACION RESPECTO A LA SITUACION
DUDOSO( ),NO( ),LIG.( ),MED.( ),INT.( )

8. DESORIENTACION RESPECTO A LA PROPIA PERSONA
DUDOSO( ),NO( ),LIG.( ),MED.( ),INT.( )

TRASTORNOS DE LA ATENCION Y MEMORIA

9. TRASTORNOS DE LA APREHENSION
DUDOSO( ),NO( ),LIG.( ),MED.( ),INT.( )

10. TRASTORNOS DE LA CONCENTRACION
DUDOSO( ),NO( ),LIG.( ),MED.( ),INT.( )

11. TRASTORNOS DE LA MEMORIA A CORTO PLAZO
DUDOSO( ),NO( ),LIG.( ),MED.( ),INT.( )

12. TRASTORNOS DE LA MEMORIA
DUDOSO( ),NO( ),LIG.( ),MED.( ),INT.( )

13. CONFABULACIONES
DUDOSO( ),NO( ),LIG.( ),MED.( ),INT.( )

14. PARAMNESIAS
DUDOSO( ),NO( ),LIG.( ),MED.( ),INT.( )

TRASTORNOS FORMALES DEL PENSAMIENTO

15. INHIBICION DEL PENSAMIENTO
DUDOSO( ),NO( ),LIG.( ),MED.( ),INT.( )

16. ENLENTECIMIENTO DEL PENSAMIENTO
DUDOSO( ),NO( ),LIG.( ),MED.( ),INT.( )

17. PENSAMIENTO DIVAGATORIO
DUDOSO( ),NO( ),LIG.( ),MED.( ),INT.( )

18. POBREZA DEL PENSAMIENTO
DUDOSO( ),NO( ),LIG.( ),MED.( ),INT.( )

19. PERSEVERACION DEL PENSAMIENTO
DUDOSO( ),NO( ),LIG.( ),MED.( ),INT.( )

20. RUMIACION
DUDOSO( ),NO( ),LIG.( ),MED.( ),INT.( )

21. ACELERACION DEL PENSAMIENTO
DUDOSO( ),NO( ),LIG.( ),MED.( ),INT.( )

22. FUGA DE IDEAS
DUDOSO( ),NO( ),LIG.( ),MED.( ),INT.( )

23. PARARRESPUESTAS
DUDOSO( ),NO( ),LIG.( ),MED.( ),INT.( )

24. BLOQUEO DEL PENSAMIENTO O INTERCEPTACION
DUDOSO( ),NO( ),LIG.( ),MED.( ),INT.( )

Subject Index

Antidepressants and neuroleptics evaluated with the help of the AMP/AMDP-System are not listed here but in the Appendix I. In italics, the pages containing a facsimile of the scales.